Review Questions for
HUMAN EMBRYOLOGY

Review Questions for
HUMAN EMBRYOLOGY

by

Thomas R. Gest, PhD
Associate Professor, Office of Educational Development
University of Arkansas for Medical Sciences

Jeffrey M. Anderson, MD
Primary Care Sports Medicine Fellow
University of Connecticut Medical Center

Review Questions Series
Series Editor: Thomas R. Gest, PhD
University of Arkansas for Medical Sciences

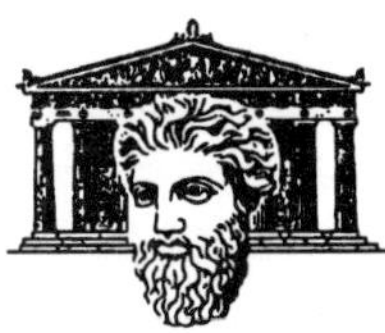

The Parthenon Publishing Group Inc.
International Publishers in Medicine, Science & Technology

One Blue Hill Plaza, Pearl River, New York 10965, USA

Published in the USA by
The Parthenon Publishing Group Inc.
One Blue Hill Plaza,
PO Box 1564, Pearl River,
New York 10965

Published in Europe by
The Parthenon Publishing Group Limited
Casterton Hall, Carnforth,
Lancs LA6 2LA, UK

Library of Congress Cataloging-in-Publication Data

Gest, Thomas R.
Review questions for human embryology / by Thomas R. Gest, Jeffrey M. Anderson.
p. cm. – (Review questions series)
ISBN: 1-85070-591-7
1. Embryology, Human – Examinations, questions, etc. I. Anderson, Jeffrey M. II. Title. III. Series.
[DNLM: 1. Embryology – examination questions. 2. Embryo – physiology – examination questions. 3. Embryo – anatomy & histology – examination questions. 4. Fetal Development – examination questions. QS 618 G393r 1995]
QM601.G47 1995
612.6′4′076 – dc20
DNLM/DLC
for Library of Congress 94-41657
CIP

British Library Cataloguing in Publication Data

Gest, Thomas R.
Review Questions for Human Embryology. – (Review Questions Series)
I. Title II. Anderson, Jeffrey, M. III. Series
612.640076
ISBN 1-85070-591-7

This edition published 1995

Printed in the United States

Acknowledgements

Many people contributed to this project, and all are owed a debt of thanks for their work and dedication. Some of these individuals were medical students who I came to know while I was on the faculty of the University of Michigan Medical School. I thank all of the medical students, from the University of Michigan and the Medical College of Georgia, who helped in the completion of this project. My intent at the beginning of this project was to create something that could help medical students through their challenging coursework, and it has been the medical students who have helped me through this challenging project.

I owe my wife, Donna, a great deal of thanks for her help throughout this project, and I would also like to thank my step-daughter, Shannon Campbell, for her help on this and other projects. Without the help and support of my family, this project never would have been completed.

Thomas R. Gest, PhD

Dedicated to all of my students,
past, present and future.

Preface

This book is designed to present the student with test questions that may give an indication of the types of questions often asked about a particular subject. Work with these questions should occur after the student has gained a firm knowledge of the material. The questions can then be used to reaffirm this knowledge and to indicate where gaps in knowledge may exist. The questions should not be used as the primary study tool, but should be used as an aid to the study of embryology.

Many of the questions found in this book have been used on examinations at a number of medical schools, including University of Pittsburgh, University of North Dakota, University of South Carolina, University of Michigan, and Medical College of Georgia. The terminology presented in the questions may differ somewhat from that which you have learned. Fortunately, embryology does not vary much from state to state, so the substance of the questions should still apply.

The questions presented in these volumes are in standard, single best answer or type A format, or in type K format. The key for type K format questions is:

Type K Key

A. 1, 2 and 3 are correct.
B. 1 and 3 are correct.
C. 2 and 4 are correct.
D. only 4 is correct.
E. all are correct.

Contents

Number in parentheses indicates number of questions available.

SECTION 1: GENERAL PRINCIPLES

1.001 Parturition divides ontogeny into a prenatal period and a postnatal period.

A. true
B. false

A. is correct.
Parturition, or childbirth, ends the 38 week period of prenatal development, or ontogeny, and begins the long postnatal period of development, sometimes made longer and more difficult by medical school.

1.002 The embryonic period begins at fertilization and ends at the end of the eighth week post-conception.

A. true
B. false

B. is correct.
The embryonic period begins at three weeks, and ends at 8 weeks. The fetal period lasts from 9 weeks until term at 38 weeks. The earliest period does not have as snappy of a name, but has been called the period of the ovum. During this period, conceptus changes from zygote to morula to blastocyst to gastrula to become embryo.

1.003 One of the characteristics of humans that complicate the act of childbirth is the relatively large head of the newborn. This is because the brain does not grow after birth.

A. true
B. false

B. is correct.
The brain will grow significantly after birth, and will triple its weight during the first two decades of life. However, what goes up must come down, and the brain actually shrinks gradually in the later years of life.

1.004 A plane passing through the body that divides the body into equal right and left halves is called a ________.

A. coronal
B. transverse
C. sagittal
D. medial
E. vertical

C. is correct.
A sagittal or median plane is a vertical plane dividing the body into right & left sides. Coronal or frontal planes are vertical, but divide body into anterior-ventral-front and posterior-dorsal-back part. Transverse planes are horizontal. Medial & lateral are relative terms; medial means closer to midline.

1.005 A developmental increase in mass is called:

A. histogenesis
B. morphogenesis
C. growth
D. proliferation
E. fertilization

C. is correct.
A developmental increase in mass is called growth. Morphogenesis is the development of form, pattern, or structure during embryonic development. Proliferation is an increase in cell number, but not necessarily in size, such as in the morula formation. Histogenesis is the differentiation of cells into tissue types.

1.006 Diversity of form is brought about by:

A. differential rates of growth
B. metaplasia
C. absolute growth
D. protoplasmic synthesis
E. none of the above

A. is correct.
Differential rates of growth of some cells and tissues result in diversity of form. Of course, histogenesis or the differentiation of tissues is important in creating a diversity of form in the developing body.

1.007 Of the following, factor(s) controlling growth is/are:

A. temperature
B. hormones
C. nutritional factors
D. heredity
E. all of the above

E. is correct.
All of the items mentioned affect the process of growth.

1.008 Specific morphogenetic processes include:

A. cell migration
B. fusion and splitting
C. folding
D. differential growth
E. all of the above

E. is correct.
According to Arey, cell migration, cell aggregation, localized growth, fusion & splitting and folding & bending are all involved in morphogenesis, or the development of form and pattern.

1.009 Select the best term describing the hand in reference to the arm:

A. ventral
B. posterior
C. inferior
D. distal
E. proximal

D. is correct.
With regard to correct anatomical position, the term "distal" refers to a position farther out along the root of a limb, which is the case with the hand in reference to the arm. Proximal means closer. Ventral is toward the front, posterior is toward the back. Inferior or caudal is down, superior or cranial is up.

1.010 In the adult, it is stated that the thorax is superior to the abdomen. The corresponding term for an embryo is:

A. dorsal
B. cranial
C. caudal
D. posterior
E. inferior

B. is correct.
Because the adult stands erect, the thorax is superior to the abdomen by virtue of its position above the abdomen. However, since the embryo does not stand erect, the correct term would be cranial because the thorax is closer to the head end of the embryo than is the abdomen.

SECTION 2: GAMETOGENESIS

2.001 Which of the following types of germ cells does not undergo cell division?

A. spermatogonia
B. primary oocytes
C. spermatids
D. secondary oocytes
E. oogonia

C. is correct.
Spermatogonia and oogonia are the primitive germ cells of each sex. Oogonia differentiate into primary oocytes, which begin the first meiotic division before birth but halt in prophase, or dictyotene, stage. The primary oocytes complete the 1st meiotic division years later at ovulation. They are then called secondary oocytes.

2.002 Oogonia are homologous to spermatogonia. Oogonia divide by mitosis during:

A. all postnatal periods
B. fetal life
C. postnatal periods after puberty
D. the reproductive period
E. none of the above

B. is correct.
Oogonia divide by mitosis throughout fetal life, although they reach a maximum number of approximately 7 million during the 5th month of development. Due to degeneration, less than 2 million primary oocytes are present at birth. Mitosis of oogonia ceases well before birth.

2.003 Prior to ejaculation, sperm are stored in the:

A. seminal vesicles
B. efferent ductules
C. epididymis
D. ejaculatory ducts
E. seminal colliculus

C. is correct.
The visit to the epididymis is very important for the spermatozoa. In the environment of the epididymis, the sperm attain their full motility.

2.004 How many sperms, approximately, are deposited in the vagina during intercourse?

A. 300 thousand
B. 3 million
C. 30 million
D. 300 million
E. 3 billion

D. is correct.
Of the nearly 300 million sperms in the 3.5ml of ejaculate, only a few hundred sperms reach the ampulla of the uterine tube, the site of fertilization. Sperm count less than 20 million per ml indicates probable sterility.

2.005 The first meiotic division of the primary oocytes is characterized by:

A. pairing of homologous chromosomes
B. DNA replication
C. crossing over
D. production of a polar body
E. all of the above

E. is correct.
The first meiotic division in female sex cells involves replication of the DNA, pairing of the homologous chromosomes and crossing over, or chiasma formation. Homologous chromosomes exchange genetic material during crossing over. Years later, at the culmination of the first meiotic division, the first polar body is given off.

2.006 The part of the sperm containing proteolytic enzymes to digest the zona pellucida is the:

A. capacitor
B. head
C. corona
D. acrosome
E. cumulus

D. is correct.
The acrosome is the part of the sperm containing proteolytic enzymes to digest the zona pellucida. It is exposed by the process of capacitation. Then, under the influence of substances released by corona radiata cells, it releases its proteolytic enzymes and penetrates the oocyte.

2.007 The ovulated mammalian oocyte is arrested at:

A. prophase of meiosis I
B. metaphase of meiosis I
C. prophase of meiosis II
D. metaphase of meiosis II
E. none of the above

D. is correct.
The long arrest in meiosis occurs in the primary oocyte. These descendants of oogonia begin meiosis before birth and stop dividing during prophase of the first division. Years later, this first division is completed just prior to ovulation. Ovulated secondary oocytes then stop at metaphase II until fertilized.

2.008 The second meiotic division differs from the first meiotic division in that:

A. crossing over only occurs during meiosis I
B. there is pairing of the homologous chromosome during meiosis I
C. there is no DNA synthesis during meiosis II
D. all of the above
E. none of the above

D. is correct.
During the first meiotic division, DNA is replicated and homologous chromosomes pair. This pair exchanges genetic material in crossing over. In meiosis II, the DNA is not replicated. Therefore, haploid chromosome number is reached.

2.009 The zona pellucida:

A. is synthesized by the oocyte during oogenesis
B. contains species-specific sperm receptor molecules
C. is modified post-fertilization to block polyspermy
D. all of the above
E. none of the above

D. is correct.
Zona pellucida, produced by the oocyte, is designed to receive only sperm of the same species. After the penetration of the first sperm through the zona, the zona reaction occurs, making zona impenetrable to other sperm. After the first sperm enters the oocyte, a cortical reaction makes its cell membrane impenetrable.

2.010 Nondisjunction is the result of an abnormal meiotic division that:

A. is thought to occur during oogenesis
B. can result in autosomal trisomy
C. can result in an individual with 47 chromosomes
D. can be the result of homologous chromosomes failing to separate
E. all of the above are correct

E. is correct.
Nondisjunction occurs during the meiotic divisions of sex cells. It occurs when homologous chromosomes fail to separate, contributing an extra chromosome to one daughter cell and one too few to the other. If the cell with the extra chromosome is fertilized, it can lead to a zygote with 47 chromosomes, or trisomy.

2.011 During gametogenesis, meiosis occurs which reduces the chromosome number from _______ to _______.

A. diploid to haploid
B. haploid to tetraploid
C. dizygotic to monozygotic
D. bicornate to unicornate
E. azygos to hemiazygos

A. is correct.
Meiosis reduces the chromosome number from diploid to haploid. The union of two haploid cells in fertilization restores the diploid state. Monozygotic twinning results from a splitting of the early ovum, while dizygotic twins result from two separate fertilizations.

2.012 The human male has how many different chromosomes?

A. 48
B. 46
C. 47
D. 24
E. 26

D. is correct.
The human male has 46 chromosomes, as does the human female. However, because chromosomes come in pairs and the male's sex chromosomes are different, X & Y, he has 24 DIFFERENT chromosomes. The human female, on the other hand, has identical sex chromosomes, two X's, giving her 23 DIFFERENT chromosomes.

2.013 As the follicle grows, the oogonium becomes located in a mound of follicle cells called the:

A. vesicular antrum
B. oocyte
C. cumulus oophorus
D. liquor folliculi
E. none of these

C. is correct.
As the antrum, or cavity, forms and enlarges within the follicle, a collection of follicular cells remain around the oocyte. These cells form a mound called the cumulus oophorus. The antrum is full of fluid called liquor folliculi. The oocyte is the female sex cell often called the egg or ovum.

2.014 How many different kinds of chromosomes are there in a human female?

A. 22
B. 23
C. 24
D. 25
E. 47

B. is correct.
The human genome consists of 23 pairs of chromosomes, 46 in all. Of these, one pair is the sex chromosomes. Because the female has identical sex chromosomes (two X's) she would only have 23 different chromosomes. The male, on the other hand, has two different sex chromosomes (X & Y) giving him 24 different chromosomes.

2.015 The secondary oocyte completes the second maturation division:

A. before ovulation
B. during ovulation
C. at fertilization
D. before birth
E. before puberty

C. is correct.
For the second maturation to be completed, fertilization must occur. Oogonia or primordial germ cells migrate into the developing ovary to become primitive oocytes by mitosis and maturation. Secondary oocytes develop from primary oocytes by completing the 1st meiotic division, which occurs just prior to ovulation.

2.016 Spermatogonia, derived from primordial germ cells, divide by mitosis during:

A. postnatal periods
B. prenatal periods
C. postnatal periods after puberty
D. the reproductive period
E. puberty

C. is correct.
Spermatogonia remain dormant in the testis until puberty, when they divide by mitosis an differentiate into either primary spermatocytes or stem cells. Stem cells continue dividing by mitosis. Primary spermatocytes undergo the 1st meiotic division to become secondary spermatocytes, then 2nd meiotic division to become spermatids.

2.017 The process of spermiogenesis involves, along with other events, the addition of a cap containing proteolytic enzymes to the head of the male sex cell. Immediately prior to spermiogenesis, the male sex cells are called _______________.

A. spermatids
B. primary oocytes
C. secondary oocytes
D. epididymis
E. acrosomes
F. spermatogonia
G. oogonia
H. cumulus oophorus
I. spermatozoa
J. polar bodies

A. is correct.
The acrosome is a cap of proteolytic enzymes which is added to the head of the spermatid during the process of spermiogenesis. With the development of other morphological features, most notably the tail, the spermatid is transformed into the sperm cell or spermatozoon.

2.018 Immediately prior to ovulation, the first meiotic division, which had been arrested in prophase I, resumes. This transforms the developing sex cells into __________________, which becomes arrested again at the second metaphase of meiosis.

A. spermatids
B. primary oocytes
C. secondary oocytes
D. epididymis
E. acrosomes
F. spermatogonia
G. oogonia
H. cumulus oophorus
I. spermatozoa
J. polar bodies

C. is correct.

During oogenesis, oogonia differentiate into primary oocytes, which initiate meiosis but become arrested at the first prophase stage. Just before ovulation, the primary oocyte resumes the meiotic division, becoming the secondary oocyte. The secondary oocyte or ovum stops meiosis again at metaphase II, and completes meiosis only if fertilized.

SECTION 3: OVULATION TO IMPLANTATION

3.001 All of the following are directly involved with the implantation process except:

A. decidual reaction
B. progesterone
C. epiblast
D. invasion
E. none of the above

C. is correct.
The decidual reaction of the endometrium creates a nourishing environment for the conceptus as it buries itself by invasion of the uterine endometrial wall. Progesterone produced by the corpus luteum stimulates glandular secretion in the endometrium during the secretory phase of menstruation or early pregnancy.

3.002 The seven-day blastocyst:

A. has a single layer of trophoblast at the embryonic pole
B. has an amniotic cavity
C. is attached to the endometrial epithelium
D. is surrounded by a degenerating zona pellucida
E. is called the hypoblast

C. is correct.
At four days, the blastocyst cavity or blastocoele forms, but the amniotic cavity does not form until early 2nd week. Zona pellucida disappears so that implantation can begin at day 6. As implantation begins, the trophoblast becomes 2 layers: syncytiotrophoblast and cytotrophoblast. Inner cell mass becomes epiblast & hypoblast.

3.003 Which of the following are classified as gonadotropin hormones?

A. FSH
B. GnRH
C. estradiol or estrogen
D. progesterone
E. all of the above

A. is correct.
Gonadotropin-releasing hormone or GnRH, from the hypothalamus, causes the anterior pituitary to secrete FSH or follicle-stimulating hormone, and LH or luteinizing hormone. These are the gonadotropins that produce the cycles of the ovary. FSH is primary in follicle development, while LH is primary in ovulation.

3.004 Haploid nuclei that fuse at fertilization are called:

A. homunculi
B. mitotic figures
C. centrioles
D. nucleoli
E. pronuclei

E. is correct.
After the sperm reaches the ovum, it deposits its genetic load, the male pronucleus, into the cytoplasm of the egg. After finally completing the meiotic division that had begun years before, the female pronucleus fuses with the male pronucleus to create the diploid nucleus of the zygote.

3.005 The first week of human development is characterized by formation of the:

A. inner cell mass
B. hypoblast
C. trophoblast
D. blastocyst
E. all of the above

E. is correct.
At four days, the blastocyst cavity or blastocele forms within the morula. Trophoblast are outer cells of the blastocyst, while a knot of cells appears, protruding into the blastocele. This is the inner cell mass. Trophoblast becomes 2 layers: syncytiotrophoblast and cytotrophoblast. Inner cell mass becomes epiblast & hypoblast.

3.006 During the follicular phase of the menstrual cycle:

A. FSH binds to the corpus luteum and stimulates estrogen production
B. FSH binds to granulosa cells of the follicle and stimulates estrogen production
C. FSH binds to the corpus luteum and stimulate progesterone production
D. FSH binds to granulosa cells of the follicle and stimulates progesterone production
E. FSH binds to granulosa cells of the follicle and stimulates LH production

B. is correct.
FSH and LH from the anterior pituitary work together toward the goal of ovulation. FSH is most important in early follicle maturation. FSH also stimulates the granulosa cells of the follicle to produce estrogen. The LH surge, caused by increased estrogen, stimulates ovulation, after which corpus luteum produces progesterone.

3.007 Gonadotropin-releasing hormone or GnRH:

A. acts on the hypothalamus, causing release of FSH & LH
B. is released once a month from the corpus luteum
C. acts on anterior pituitary gland, causing release of FSH & LH
D. acts on the anterior pituitary causing release of estrogen and progesterone
E. is one of those meaningless substances that scientists play with in lieu of working for a living

C. is correct.
GnRH is released from the hypothalamus, and stimulates the anterior pituitary to release FSH, or follicle-stimulating hormone, and LH, or luteinizing hormone. FSH & LH work together to produce ovulation and completion of the reproductive cycle.

3.008 The LH surge:

A. results in ovulation
B. triggers resumption of meiosis within the oocyte
C. is caused by a positive feedback effect of estrogen
D. all of the above
E. none of the above

D. is correct.
FSH stimulates the maturation of the follicle and causes release of estrogen by the granulosa cells of the follicle. The increase in estrogen induces the LH surge, which causes ovulation and the completion of the first meiotic division by the primary oocyte. The primary oocyte is arrested for years in the first prophase.

3.009 The luteal/progestational/secretory phase of the menstrual cycle is characterized by:

A. high circulating levels of FSH and LH
B. high circulating levels of progesterone
C. an extreme variation in length from cycle to cycle
D. a thin, non-vascularized endometrium
E. none of the above

B. is correct.
After the proliferative/follicular phase which culminates in ovulation, the secretory phase begins. Progesterone from the corpus luteum reaches its peak, and it acts to prepare a thick endometrial lining for possible implantation which should occur at day 20. If fertilization does not occur, endometrium becomes ischemic.

3.010 The second polar body:

A. is released upon stimulation of the follicle by FSH
B. is released as a result of the LH surge
C. is released after fertilization
D. is released after pronuclear formation
E. is also known as the south pole

C. is correct.
After the sperm has entered the oocyte and triggered the zona and cortical reactions to prevent polyspermy, the secondary oocyte completes the second meiotic division which began at ovulation. The second polar body is given off, and the male and female pronuclei fuse to form the diploid zygote nucleus.

3.011 The corpus luteum:

A. is only functional during the follicular phase of the menstrual cycle
B. has receptors for progesterone and estrogen
C. is rescued from decline by hCG secreted by the implanted embryo
D. produces both FSH and LH
E. none of the above

C. is correct.
Syncytiotrophoblast secretes hCG or human chorionic gonadotropin. Under hCG influence, corpus luteum does not decline to become the corpus albicans, but is maintained as the corpus luteum of pregnancy which secretes, as before, progesterone and estrogen. Corpus luteum is active in this role through the first half of pregnancy.

3.012 During implantation, the blastocyst:

A. implants in the endometrium
B. usually attaches to endometrial epithelium at its embryonic pole
C. usually implants in the posterior wall of the body of the uterus
D. causes change in the endometrial tissues
E. all of the above are correct

E. is correct.
Implantation occurs when the trophoblast cells at the embryonic pole secrete proteolytic enzymes that allow the blastocyst to penetrate the wall of the uterus, usually the posterior wall. The endometrial lining responds to implantation through the decidua reaction, by which it becomes more succulent for nourishing the blastocyst.

3.013 Capacitation of the sperm:

A. is caused by the zona pellucida
B. occurs in the male
C. prevents polyspermy
D. is essential for fertilization
E. removes the head of the sperm

D. is correct.
Capacitation involves removing the glycoprotein coat and seminal plasma proteins from the head of the sperm, exposing the acrosome and allowing the acrosome reaction to occur. Capacitation occurs within the female genital tract, and without its occurrence, fertilization could not occur.

3.014 The most significant factors in sperm transport to the vicinity of the oocyte is:

A. sperm flagellum (tail)
B. vaginal cilia
C. an intact zona pellucida
D. smooth muscle contractions
E. gravity

D. is correct.
The most important contributors to sperm transport within the female genital tract are oviductal cilia and smooth muscle contractions. The sperm flagellum is most useful very close to the ovum, and an intact zona pellucida is essential, because the zona reaction occurs after the first sperm passage, making zona impenetrable.

3.015 The early stages of cleavage are characterized by:

A. formation of a hollow ball of cells
B. formation of the zona pellucida
C. increase in the size of the cells in the zygote
D. increase in the number of cells in the zygote
E. none of the above

D. is correct.
The earliest stages of cleavage are marked by a series of mitotic divisions that increase the number of cells in the zygote without an increase in size. As the cleavage continues the zygote becomes a morula or a solid ball of 12-16 cells. A cavity forming within the morula transforms it into a blastocyst, at about day 4.

3.016 The most common site for implantation in ectopic pregnancy is:

A. internal os of the uterus
B. mesentery
C. ovary
D. uterine tube
E. other

D. is correct.
The most common site of ectopic implantation is the uterine tube. The growth of the embryo in this site usually causes rupture of the tube and severe hemorrhage in the mother. Abdominally, an ectopic pregnancy often occurs in the rectouterine pouch, an area between the uterus and the rectum.

3.017 During the morula stage:

A. tight junctions appear between peripheral cells, isolating the inner cells from uterine fluid
B. the location of the cells dictates their fate
C. the outer cells pump fluid, creating a fluid-filled blastocoele
D. attachment to the uterine epithelium has not yet occurred
E. all of the above are correct

E. is correct.
The morula is composed of inner cells and a layer of surrounding cells, which differentiate along different lines. Although there are tight junctions between the outer cells, they pump fluid in, forming the blastocoele. The embryo does not implant until it reaches the blastocyst stage.

3.018 Capacitation of spermatozoa is an activation process that involves changes in the surface coat and plasma membrane over the ________.

A. tail
B. body
C. neck
D. acrosome
E. nucleus

D. is correct.
During capacitation, the glycoprotein coat and seminal plasma proteins are removed from the plasma membrane overlying the acrosome. This exposes the acrosome and allows the acrosome reaction to occur.

3.019 Implantation will not take place unless the zona ________ is lost.

A. pellucida
B. limitans
C. orbicularis
D. corona
E. oophorus

A. is correct.
The zona pellucida disappears around the end of the fourth day. It is not possible for implantation to occur until it is lost.

3.020 The results of fertilization include the determination of chromosomal sex and initiation of cleavage.

A. true
B. false

A. is correct.
At fertilization, you have the restoration of a diploid number of chromosomes, the determination of sex and the initiation of cleavage. Sex is determined by the sperm, which carries either an X or a Y chromosome. All oocytes contain an X sex chromosome.

3.021 Before a spermatozoan can fertilize an ovum:

A. the cell membrane is removed from the spermatozoan head
B. the zona pellucida must be shed
C. the acrosomal membrane must perforate
D. the tailpiece is lost
E. the decidua reaction must occur

C. is correct.
Capacitation, in which a glycoprotein coat is shed from the sperm head, and the acrosome reaction, in which the acrosomal membrane perforates, must occur for fertilization to take place. Zona pellucida is not lost until after the fourth day of development. Decidua reaction occurs after fertilization.

3.022 At fertilization:

A. the haploid number of chromosomes is restored
B. the chromosomal sex is determined
C. cleavage is inhibited
D. the inner cell mass becomes recognizable
E. the ovum becomes the blastocyst

B. is correct.
At fertilization, you have the restoration of a diploid number of chromosomes, the determination of sex and the initiation of cleavage. The inner cell mass does not become recognizable until the blastocyst stage, at day 4.

3.023 Which of the following events are directly related to implantation?

A. interaction between uterine endometrium and hypoblast
B. release of proteolytic enzymes
C. loss of the decidua
D. acrosome reaction
E. capacitation

B. is correct.
When the zona pellucida is lost, the blastocyst is able to release proteolytic enzymes that allow it to penetrate the uterine wall. The uterine mucosal lining also aids in promoting enzyme release. The acrosome reaction is not related to implantation in that it occurs before fertilization.

3.024 In ectopic pregnancy:

A. the placenta overbridges the internal os of the uterus
B. implantation is inside the uterus
C. severe bleeding is present during vaginal delivery
D. the most common site is the uterine tube

D. is correct.
Ectopic pregnancy implies implantation at some site other than the uterus. The most common site is the oviduct. When the placenta overbridges the uterine internal os, it called placenta previa, and can cause massive bleeding at delivery.

3.025 Approximately how many million sperm are there in the average ejaculate of 3.5 cc?

A. 5
B. 50
C. 100
D. 200
E. more than 200

E. is correct.
There are more than 200 million sperm in the average ejaculate. A better question is: who counted all those sperm, and why?

3.026 The meeting and union of human sex cells is believed to occur in the:

A. upper third of the oviduct
B. middle third of the oviduct
C. lower third of the oviduct
D. uterus
E. cervix

A. is correct.
Fertilization occurs in the upper third of uterine tube, a region called the ampullary region. The sperm are transported there primarily by muscular contractions and by action of the cilia in the uterine tube.

3.027 Sexuality is established at the time of:

A. ovulation
B. gametogenesis
C. histogenesis
D. morphogenesis
E. none of the above

E. is correct.
Sexuality is determined at the time of fertilization, so none of the answers are correct.

3.028 Cleavage divisions are always:

A. meiotic
B. mitotic
C. amniotic
D. anucleotic
E. by binary fission

B. is correct.
The divisions that occur during cleavage are always mitotic, producing daughter cells with a diploid number of chromosomes. However, in cleavage there is no period of cell growth between divisions, so that the originally oversized ovum is fractionalized through cleavage into cells, called blastomeres, of normal size.

3.029 At which of the following stages of development is division of embryonic material likely to result in normal monozygotic twinning?

A. 2-cell stage
B. morula
C. blastocyst
D. implanting embryo
E. all of the above

E. is correct.
Splitting of the zygote can occur at any stage from the two-cell stage until the stage of the bilaminar germ disc. The splitting usually occurs at the early blastocyst stage. In this case, the inner cell mass or embryoblast splits, but they both share a common blastocoele. They will share the placenta but have separate amnions.

3.030 Ectopic implantations occur most commonly in the:

A. ovary
B. abdomen
C. uterine tube
D. cervix
E. posterior wall of the uterus

C. is correct.
The most common site of ectopic implantation is the uterine tube. The growth of the embryo in this site usually causes rupture of the tube and severe hemorrhage in the mother. Abdominally, an ectopic pregnancy often occurs in the rectouterine pouch, an area between the uterus and the rectum.

3.031 With the light microscope, the zona pellucida appears as a translucent membrane surrounding the:

A. primary oocyte
B. zygote
C. morula
D. very early blastocyst
E. all of the above are correct

E. is correct.
The zona pellucida persists until early in the blastocyst stage. It dissolves during the blastocyst stage in order that implantation may occur.

3.032 The fifth day of human development is characterized by embryonic cells of the:

A. inner cell mass
B. embryonic hypoblast
C. epiblast
D. primitive streak
E. amnion

A. is correct.
By the fifth day, the blastocyst has developed an inner cell mass or embryoblast and an outer trophoblast. However, the inner cell mass has not yet divided into an epiblast and hypoblast. The primitive streak does not form until the third week.

3.033 The _______ is/are part(s) of the 4-day blastocyst:

A. syncytiotrophoblast
B. blastocyst cavity
C. notochord
D. somitomeres

B. is correct.
It is still too early for the syncytiotrophoblast (day 7-8) and the notochord (week 3) to be present, but the blastocyst cavity is present as are blastomeres, the cells that make up the blastocyst.

3.034 It is approximately correct to compute the age of an embryo from the fourteenth day after:

A. onset of last menstruation
B. last sexual intercourse
C. last full moon
D. last missed menstrual period
E. onset of breast changes

A. is correct.
Since ovulation, and hence, fertilization occur about fourteen days after the onset of the last menstruation, it would be fairly accurate to compute the age of an embryo in that manner. It is true that full moons are romantic, though, and sexual intercourse seems to have a great deal to do with conception.

3.035 As the conceptus begins to sink into the uterine lining, it is characterized by a central cavity surrounded for the most part by a single layer of cells. At this stage the conceptus is called a ________________.

A. zygote
B. morula
C. blastocyst
D. trophoblast
E. syncytiotrophoblast
F. cytotrophoblast
G. blastocoele
H. inner cell mass
I. blastomere
J. embryoblast
K. zona pellucida

C. is correct.
The blastocyst cavity or blastocoele forms within the solid ball of cells called the morula, transforming it into the blastocyst. The single layer of cells surrounding the blastocoele is the trophoblast, which differentiates into an outer syncytiotrophoblast and an inner cytotrophoblast.

SECTION 4: SECOND AND THIRD WEEKS

4.001 The completion of interstitial implantation, so that the conceptus is entirely within the endometrium, occurs:

A. on about day 20
B. by about day 11
C. by the end of the first week
D. by erosion of the myometrial lining
E. as a result of endodermal proliferation

B. is correct.
The blastocyst attaches to the endometrium of the uterine wall, usually posterior wall, on day 6. Implantation proceeds until about day 10-11 when the defect in the endometrium where the blastocyst implanted is covered by a closing plug.

4.002 Both the neurenteric canal and the notochordal plate are present in the conceptus at the same time.

A. true
B. false

A. is correct.
When the floor of the notochordal process disappears, forming the notochordal plate, a temporary communication is opened between the amniotic cavity and the yolk sac. This opening is the neurenteric canal. Notochordal plate forms the definitive notochord, which will induce neural tube formation.

4.003 Much of the intraembryonic coelom forms within paraxial mesoderm.

A. true
B. false

B. is correct.
The intraembryonic coelom forms within the lateral or lateral plate mesoderm. Paraxial mesoderm is the somitic mesoderm lying adjacent to the notochord. Intermediate mesoderm lies between lateral and paraxial mesoderm.

4.004 The amniotic cavity develops:

A. on the tenth day
B. within the outer cell mass
C. within the inner cell mass near the cytotrophoblast
D. in extraembryonic mesoderm
E. none of the above

C. is correct.
The amniotic cavity begins to develop around the 8th day as a slit-like area within the epiblast near the cytotrophoblast. It usually has a thin strip of epiblast cells, called amnioblasts, between it and the cytotrophoblast.

4.005 During the second week of development, the trophoblast differentiates into:

A. syncytiotrophoblast
B. ectoderm
C. intraembryonic mesoderm
D. yolk sac (secondary)

A. is correct.
The trophoblast gives rise to both the syncytiotrophoblast and the cytotrophoblast, as well as the extraembryonic mesoderm. The ectoderm is a derivative of the epiblast, and the secondary yolk sac comes from endoderm cells that line the exocoelomic cavity or the primitive yolk sac.

4.006 Major events beginning in the second week of development include:

A. notochord differentiation
B. somite formation
C. angiogenesis
D. yolk sac development

D. is correct.
Yolk sac development is the only item mentioned that occurs as early as the second week. Notochord differentiation, somite formation and angiogenesis do not begin until the third week.

4.007 The first two intraembryonic germ layers to differentiate are the:

A. ectoderm & hypoblast
B. epiblast & hypoblast
C. ectoderm & endoderm
D. ectoderm & mesoderm

B. is correct.
The epiblast & hypoblast develop from the inner cell mass during the 2nd week. During the 3rd week, the epiblast produces cells between itself and the hypoblast, called the mesoderm. Epiblast also replaces the hypoblast with endoderm cells. Epiblast then changes its name to ectoderm, completing the process of gastrulation.

4.008 The blastocoele becomes the:

A. amniotic cavity
B. extraembryonic coelom
C. primary yolk sac
D. chorionic cavity
E. secondary cavity

C. is correct.
Around the 9th day, cells from the hypoblast spread around the blastocoele, forming the exocoelomic or Heuser's membrane. When the blastocoele is surrounded by this membrane, it is referred to as the primary yolk sac or exocoelomic cavity.

4.009 Extraembryonic somatic mesoderm is in close association with:

A. syncytiotrophoblast
B. cytotrophoblast & amnion
C. yolk sac
D. syncytio- & cytotrophoblast

B. is correct.
Extraembryonic mesoderm arises from the cytotrophoblast. The extraembryonic SOMATIC mesoderm lines the cytotrophoblast and the amnion. The extraembryonic SPLANCHNIC mesoderm lines the yolk sac. The syncytiotrophoblast is separated from the extraembryonic somatic mesoderm by the cytotrophoblast.

4.010 Cytotrophoblast cells become:

A. secondary yolk sac
B. amnioblasts
C. exocoelomic membrane
D. syncytiotrophoblast

D. is correct.
The cytotrophoblast cells can differentiate into syncytiotrophoblast cells. However, the secondary yolk sac is from endoderm, the amnioblasts are from epiblast, and the exocoelomic membrane is from hypoblast.

4.011 The yolk sac in the human embryo:

A. does not contribute to the embryonic gut
B. is devoid of hemopoietic activity, or blood cell formation
C. is the site of primordial germ cell production
D. stores nutrients throughout pregnancy

C. is correct.
The definitive yolk sac, which forms at the end of the 2nd week, serves many purposes in the developing embryo. Its endodermal lining becomes the lining of the embryonic gut. Blood islands form within its wall. It is also the site of primordial germ cell production. It has little nutritional role in humans, though.

4.012 The bilaminar germ disc:

A. consists of epiblast and mesoblast
B. is derived from the outer cells of the morula
C. forms the embryo proper
D. synthesizes human chorionic gonadotropin, HCG

C. is correct.
The bilaminar germ disc develops from the inner cells of the morula and inner cell mass of the blastocyst. It is composed of epiblast & hypoblast layers, and it is also called the embryoblast because it becomes the embryo. The outer cells of the morula & blastocyst become cyto- & syncytiotrophoblast. The latter produces HCG.

4.013 The definitive yolk sac of the embryo appears by what day?

A. 13th
B. 26th
C. 72nd
D. 94th
E. 2nd

A. is correct.
Around the 13th day, the definitive yolk sac is formed by the hypoblast cells that line the inside of the exocoelomic membrane.

4.014 The amniotic cavity appears as a slit-like space near the embryonic polar trophoblast and within the:

A. extraembryonic mesoderm
B. exocoelomic membrane
C. inner cell mass
D. connecting body stalk
E. cytotrophoblast

C. is correct.
The amniotic cavity begins to appear around the eighth day of development within the inner cell mass adjacent to the embryonic pole. The cells that line this cavity are called amnioblasts, and they form the amnion.

4.015 During the second week, the embryonic disk is composed of:

A. ectoderm
B. ectoderm and mesoderm
C. endoderm
D. epiblast and hypoblast
E. ectoderm, mesoderm and endoderm

D. is correct.
In the second week, you still have a bilaminar germ disc because the primitive streak has not yet formed, allowing for invagination and the formation of the mesoderm. This occurs during the third week. In the bilaminar germ disc, the correct terminology for the two layers is epiblast and hypoblast.

4.016 The part of the 13-day embryoblast from which the embryo proper is formed:

A. lies between the amniotic cavity and yolk sac
B. also contributes to the roof of the yolk sac
C. is composed of two primary germ layers
D. is attached to the amnion
E. all of the above are correct

E. is correct.
The epiblast and hypoblast, from which the embryo comes, lie between the amniotic cavity and the yolk sac, to which the hypoblast contributes the roof. Since invagination has yet to occur, there are still only two primary germ layers. Amnion attaches to or is continuous with the margins of the epiblast layer of the disc.

4.017 The cloacal membrane consists of:

A. embryonic endoderm, mesoderm and ectoderm
B. endoderm of the roof of the yolk sac and embryonic ectoderm
C. a spherical area of endoderm fused to embryonic mesoderm
D. the prochordal plate and the overlying embryonic endoderm
E. none of the above

B. is correct.
Once the mesodermal layer has formed, the only places at which the ectoderm and endoderm are in direct apposition are the prochordal plate cranially and the cloacal membrane caudally. In these areas, the embryonic ectoderm is fused with the endoderm of the roof of the yolk sac.

4.018 The amniotic cavity develops:

A. on the 10th day
B. within the inner cell mass
C. between inner cell mass and trophoblast
D. in the extraembryonic mesoderm
E. between two layers of cytotrophoblast

C. is correct.
Different authors offer slightly different interpretations of the position of the amniotic cavity formation. Some place it between inner cell mass and cytotrophoblast, while others place it within the epiblast. This distinction rests on the interpretation of the origin of the amnioblasts, either from cytotrophoblast or epiblast.

4.019 Which statement about the 14-day blastocyst is NOT true?

A. villi are absent
B. extraembryonic coelom surrounds the yolk sac
C. primitive uteroplacental circulation is established
D. extraembryonic mesoderm is split into two layers
E. none of the above

A. is correct.
Syncytiotrophoblast extends processes into endometrium at the end of the 1st week, and spaces called lacunae or sinusoids appear within this syncytium during the 2nd week. Maternal blood leaking into the lacunae initiates uteroplacental circulation. Primary villi form near 2 weeks as cytotrophoblast invades syncytium.

4.020 The primitive streak first appears at the beginning of the ___ week.

A. first
B. second
C. third
D. fourth
E. fifth

C. is correct.
Gastrulation, the process of formation of the three germ layers, occurs during the third week. Epiblast cells form a thickening called the primitive streak, with a primitive knot or node located at its cranial end. Epiblast cells invaginate from this streak to form the mesoderm layer and to replace hypoblast with endoderm.

4.021 Which of the following structures is believed to be a primary organizer or inducer during organogenesis?

A. somites
B. notochord
C. metanephric blastema
D. lens placode
E. none of the above

B. is correct.
The notochord is thought to be an important structure in induction of nervous system development, axial skeleton development and other organogenic events.

4.022 Cells from the primitive streak DO NOT become:

A. endoderm
B. intermediate mesoderm
C. paraxial mesoderm
D. lateral plate mesoderm
E. amnioblasts

E. is correct.
All mesoderm is a derivative of the invaginating cells at the primitive streak. The invagination occurs at the beginning of the third week. It is interesting that endoderm cells are also derived from the epiblast during gastrulation, replacing the hypoblast.

4.023 The primitive streak:

A. is derived from the outer cells of the morula
B. is formed during the second week in development
C. persists as the cloacal membrane
D. is the site of involution of epiblast cells to form mesoderm
E. was done in a bathing suit, for those who remember streaking

D. is correct.
The primitive streak begins to form on the surface of the epiblast at the beginning of the third week. It is at the primitive streak that epiblast cells invaginate to form the mesoderm, through the process of gastrulation. Streaking was a fad of the 1970's that involved running naked in public, definitely not a winter sport.

4.024 Teratomas are:

A. the product of teratogens
B. malformed fetuses
C. a type of tumor containing tissue from all germ layers
D. derived from trophoblast
E. none of the above

C. is correct.
Teratomas are a type of tumor containing tissue from all germ layers. These tumors often arise from persistent remnants of the primitive streak and are often found in the sacrococcygeal area. Other teratomas, that are not derivatives of the primitive streak, can be found in the ovaries and testes.

4.025 Identify the correct association:

A. adrenal cortex - ectoderm
B. blood vessels of the stomach - endoderm
C. lung epithelium - mesoderm
D. olfactory epithelium - brain
E. liver parenchyma (functional cells) - endoderm

E. is correct.
Of those structures mentioned, the adrenal cortex and blood vessels of the stomach are mesodermal. The lung epithelium and liver parenchyma are endodermal, and the olfactory epithelium is ectodermal.

4.026 In the third week of human embryonic development:

A. the amnion appears
B. a bilaminar embryonic disc is formed
C. the body stalk moves ventrally and joins with the yolk sac stalk to form the umbilical cord
D. the neural plate is induced by the notochordal process and associated mesoderm
E. the uteroplacental circulation is established

D. is correct.
It is during the third week that the notochordal process and its associated mesoderm induce the neural plate. The hollow notochordal process eventually becomes the solid notochord, the forerunner of the axial skeleton.

4.027 During development, the notochordal process:

A. arises from involuting endodermal cells
B. extends from the prochordal plate to the primitive node
C. is involved in the induction of the primitive gut
D. becomes the appendicular skeleton

B. is correct.
The notochordal process extends from the primitive node up to the prochordal plate. It develops into the notochord, around which the vertebral column forms. The notochord is not endodermal, and does not induce the primitive gut. It persists in the adult only as the nucleus pulposus of the intervertebral discs.

4.028 At the caudal end of the primitive streak, ectoderm and endoderm fuse as the:

A. notochordal canal
B. coelom
C. cloacal membrane
D. neural groove
E. notochord

C. is correct.
The ectoderm and endoderm become completely separated in the trilaminar germ disc, except at two points. The cranial fusion of the two germ layers is the prochordal plate, and the caudal fusion is the cloacal membrane.

4.029 Intraembryonic mesoderm differentiates into the:

A. yolk sac
B. neural tube
C. intermediate mesoderm
D. primordial germ cells

C. is correct.
The intraembryonic mesoderm differentiates into somites, intermediate mesoderm and lateral plate mesoderm. The neural tube is ectodermal in origin, and the primary germ cells arise from the endoderm of the yolk sac.

4.030 The lining of the ____________ forms the lining of the embryonic gut.

A. ectoderm
B. hypoblast
C. blastocyst
D. trophoblast
E. syncytiotrophoblast
F. cytotrophoblast
G. blastocoele
H. inner cell mass
I. notochord
J. extraembryonic mesoderm
K. primary yolk sac
L. amniotic cavity
M. intraembryonic coelom
N. secondary yolk sac

N. is correct.
The lining of the gut is derived from the endodermal lining of the secondary yolk sac.

4.031 The __________ gives rise to the extraembryoinc mesoderm.

A. ectoderm
B. hypoblast
C. blastocyst
D. trophoblast
E. syncytiotrophoblast
F. cytotrophoblast
G. blastocoele
H. inner cell mass
I. notochord
J. prochordal plate
K. primary yolk sac
L. amniotic cavity
M. intraembryonic coelom
N. secondary yolk sac

F. is correct.
The inner layer of the trophoblast is the cytotrophoblast. It gives rise to the extraembryonic mesoderm which surrounds the endodermal lining of the yolk sac. The extraembryonic mesoderm is split into splanchnic and somatic layers by the formation of the extraembryonic coelom or chorionic cavity.

4.032 Which layer of the bilaminar embryonic disc forms part of the lining of the amniotic cavity?

A. epiblast
B. hypoblast
C. blastocyst
D. trophoblast
E. syncytiotrophoblast
F. cytotrophoblast
G. blastocoele
H. inner cell mass
I. notochord
J. prochordal plate
K. primary yolk sac
L. amnioblast
M. intraembryonic coelom
N. secondary yolk sac

A. is correct.
The bilaminar embryonic disc comprises the epiblast and the hypoblast. Epiblast forms part of the lining of the amniotic cavity, while the hypoblast lines part of the primitive yolk sac.

SECTION 5: EMBRYONIC AND FETAL PERIODS

5.001 All of the essential features of external body form are completed by the end of the ____ week.

A. third
B. fourth
C. fifth
D. sixth
E. eighth

E. is correct.
At the end of the embryonic period, eight weeks post-conception, the essential body structures have formed. The succeeding fetal period is primarily a period of growth and maturation.

5.002 "Quickening" or the period when fetal movements are commonly first felt by the mother occurs:

A. near the end of the first trimester
B. around the middle of the second trimester
C. at the end of the second trimester
D. at the end of the embryonic period
E. at the end of the fetal period

B. is correct.
Although reflexive fetal movements begin at the end of the first trimester, they typically cannot be felt until the fifth month of pregnancy. At the end of the fetal period, there is much movement, all of it extra-uterine.

5.003 Mesoderm lateral to the notochord:

A. is derived from hypoblast
B. differentiates into ganglia
C. migrates cranial to prochordal plate
D. induces endoderm differentiation

C. is correct.
The mesoderm lateral to the notochord arises from invagination of the epiblast at the primitive streak during the third week. Some of this mesoderm forms angiogenic clusters and migrates cranially to reach the cardiogenic area in front of the prochordal plate. Ganglia are from neural crest, which is ectodermal.

5.004 The following organs are derived from mesoderm EXCEPT:

A. skeletal musculature
B. musculature of blood vessels
C. cardiac musculature
D. suprarenal cortex
E. suprarenal medulla

E. is correct.
The suprarenal or adrenal medulla is actually a part of the sympathetic nervous system. Therefore, it is a derivative of neural crest cells, and neural crest cells are ectodermal in origin.

5.005 Paraxial (somitic) mesoderm gives rise to:

A. muscle in the stomach
B. vertebrae
C. muscles of mastication
D. skeletal muscle in the trunk and extremities
E. more than one of the above

E. is correct.
Somitic mesoderm forms the segmental mesodermal structures such as vertebrae and the musculature of the trunk and the extremities. The wall of the gut is formed by the visceral layer of mesoderm from the lateral plate mesoderm. Muscles of mastication arise from the first pharyngeal arch.

5.006 The endodermal germ layer gives rise to the epithelium and wall of the gastrointestinal tract.

A. true
B. false

B. is correct.
The epithelium of the gastrointestinal tract is, indeed, endodermal, but the wall of the tract arises from the visceral or splanchnic layer of the lateral plate mesoderm.

5.007 During the fourth week in development, the growth of head, tail and lateral folds transform the flat germ disc into a tubular embryo.

A. true
B. false

A. is correct.
It is during the fourth week that folding in the head and tail region, as well as lateral folding, transforms the trilaminar germ disc to a tubular embryo.

5.008 Somites:

A. differentiate into myotomes which give rise to skeletal muscle in trunk and limbs
B. differentiate into sclerotomes which give rise to vertebrae
C. arise from segmentation of the paraxial mesoderm
D. differentiate into myotomes which give rise to skeletal muscle of the limbs
E. all of the above are correct

E. is correct.
Somites differentiate into sclerotomes, myotomes and dermatomes. The sclerotomes give rise to the vertebrae. The myotomes give rise to skeletal muscle of the trunk and limbs. The dermatomes give rise to the dermal skin component. The skeletal muscle of the face arises from the pharyngeal arches.

5.009 Following are four structures together with a germ layer. Identify the INCORRECT association:

A. epithelium of pancreas - endoderm
B. hair - ectoderm
C. bone - mesoderm
D. heart - mesoderm
E. epithelium of lung - mesoderm

E. is correct.
The epithelium of pancreas and lung is endodermal, indicating origin from the primitive gut. Hair is ectodermal in origin. Bone arises primarily from mesoderm, although there is neural crest contribution to the bone of the face. Heart is mesodermal also.

5.010 Of the following, which is derived from endoderm?

A. muscle
B. kidney
C. gonads
D. tonsils
E. hair

D. is correct.
Tonsils arise from endodermal epithelium lining the 2nd pharyngeal pouch. Kidneys & gonads arise from intermediate mesoderm. Hair is ectodermal. Skeletal muscle is from somites and somitomeres. Cardiac & most smooth muscle is from splanchnic mesoderm. Neural crest develops some vascular smooth muscle.

5.011 Which of the following structures is NOT derived from mesenchyme?

A. muscle fiber
B. cartilage of the limbs
C. white blood cell precursor
D. epidermis
E. blood vessel

D. is correct.
Mesenchyme is a term used interchangeably with mesoderm, which forms many structures, including muscle, cartilage, blood cells and blood vessels. Epidermis, on the other hand, is of ectodermal origin, not mesenchyme. Realize, though, that the dermis, just below the epidermis, is of mesenchymal origin.

5.012 Of the following, which is derived from endoderm?

A. hypophysis
B. epithelium of pharynx
C. epithelium of anal canal
D. enamel of the teeth
E. muscle

B. is correct.
The epithelium of the pharynx is epithelium that is derived from the endodermal epithelium of the primitive gut. The epithelium of the lower part of the anal canal is derived from ectoderm, while the upper part is lined with endoderm. The boundary between endodermal and ectodermal lining is called the pectinate line.

5.013 During the period of development of the major organ systems, development and differentiation appear first in what region?

A. head
B. tail
C. mid-embryo
D. distal third
E. mid-third

A. is correct.
In the development of the cardiovascular, nervous, digestive and musculoskeletal systems, differentiation generally occurs in a cranial to caudal progression.

5.014 At the beginning of the fourth week, day 22, there are about 7-10 somites present. About how many are there at the end of the fourth week, day 28?

A. 7-10
B. 10-13
C. 20-23
D. 26-29
E. 42-44

D. is correct.
Throughout the fourth and fifth weeks of development, the number of somites in the embryo is constantly increasing. Therefore, during this period, developmental age can be expressed by the number of somites. At the end of the fourth week, the corresponding number of somites is about 26-29.

5.015 Almost all of the internal organs are well laid down at _________ months.

A. 1
B. 2
C. 3
D. 4
E. 5

B. is correct.
By the end of the embryonic period at about two months of the development almost all of the internal organs are well established. This is important, in that most malformations occur within the first two months, while the internal organs are being formed. The rest of the gestational period allows for growth and maturation.

5.016 The space between the split layers of mesoderm is the:

A. amniotic cavity
B. blastocele
C. foregut
D. hindgut
E. none of the above

E. is correct.
As the lateral plate mesoderm splits into a parietal mesoderm layer and a visceral mesoderm layer, a cavity called the intraembryonic coelom is formed. This cavity is ultimately divided into the pericardial, pleural and peritoneal cavities.

5.017 Which of the following are NOT distinctive characteristics of the fourth week of development?

A. neuropores
B. somites
C. branchial arches
D. lower limb buds
E. hand plates

E. is correct.
Flattening of the distal ends of the limb bud, or formation of hand and foot plates, usually occurs in the 6th week of development. All of the other items are characteristic of the 4th week of development.

5.018 During human embryonic development:

A. the inner cell mass develops into the fetal portion of the placenta
B. the yolk sac stores nutrients for the first four weeks of development
C. the allantois stores waste products
D. the location of cells in the morula dictates their fate

D. is correct.
The inner cell mass becomes the embryo proper. The yolk sac, in humans, has no nutritive role as it does in other animals. Although the allantois serves for waste storage in other animals, it is rudimentary in man. Basically, the ultimate fate of the cells in the morula depends upon their location.

5.019 Which of the following structures does not turn under onto the ventral surface of the embryo during folding of the head?

A. prochordal plate
B. heart
C. notochord
D. pericardial cavity
E. septum transversum

C. is correct.
The buccopharyngeal membrane, heart, pericardial cavity and septum transversum all end up as ventral structures in the embryo, whereas the notochord remains dorsal. Remember, though, that before the folding of the embryo, the heart begins its development extraembryonically in a region anterior to the prochordal plate.

5.020 At birth, the crown-rump length of the newborn averages _______ cm.

A. 19
B. 28
C. 35
D. 44
E. 52

C. is correct.
The crown-rump length of the fetus measures its sitting height. This measurement can then be correlated with the age of the fetus. Most of the fetal growth in length occurs early in the fetal period, whereas most of its growth in weight occurs late in the fetal period. The average crown-rump length at birth is 35 cm.

5.021 The embryo is called a fetus after the:

A. third week
B. second month
C. third month
D. fourth month
E. sixth month

B. is correct.
The fetal period begins after the second month or ninth week, when most of the internal organs have formed. The fetal period lasts until birth. This period is characterized by maturation and growth of the fetus.

5.022 Lanugo covers the body, some head hairs show, and fetal movements are felt by the mother when the fetus is about how many months old?

A. 5
B. 6
C. 7
D. 8
E. 9

A. is correct.
Around the fifth month, there is some head hair on the fetus, the body is covered with fine lanugo hair, and fetal movements can be readily detected by the mother. Slightly later, the skin acquires a greasy, whitish film called vernix caseosa, that may protect the fetal skin from maceration by the amniotic fluid.

5.023 Which of the following statements about fetal age and weight shows a normal relationship?

A. 8 weeks - 10 gm.
B. 12 weeks - 200 gm.
C. 20 weeks - 800 gm.
D. 26 weeks - 1000 gm.
E. 38 weeks - 4600 gm.

D. is correct.
At 26 weeks, the fetus weighs about 1000gm. The fact that a full-term, 40-week fetus weighs between 3000 and 3400gm illustrates that a great deal of fetal weight gain occurs at the end of gestation. This is in contrast to growth in length which occurs earlier in gestation.

5.024 Which of the following structures is derived from paraxial mesoderm of the cervical region?

A. enamel of the teeth
B. smooth muscle of the gut
C. mucous lining of the larynx
D. sympathetic chain ganglia
E. ureter
F. suprarenal medulla
G. patella
H. skeletal muscle of the upper limb
I. heart
J. lining of the lungs
K. spinal cord
L. parenchyma of the pancreas
M. eleventh thoracic vertebra
N. aortic arch

H. is correct.
Paraxial mesoderm forms the somites, which give rise to the axial skeleton and connective tissues of the trunk, all skeletal muscle, and the dermis. In the lower cervical regions, the somitic myotomes form the skeletal muscle of the developing upper limb. The eleventh thoracic vertebra is sclerotomal (somitic), but from lower thoracic levels.

5.025 Which of the following is derived from the splanchnic layer of the lateral plate mesoderm?

A. enamel of the teeth
B. smooth muscle of the gut
C. mucous lining of the larynx
D. sympathetic chain ganglia
E. ureter
F. suprarenal medulla
G. patella
H. skeletal muscle of the upper limb
I. parietal peritoneum
J. lining of the lungs
K. spinal cord
L. parenchyma of the pancreas
M. eleventh thoracic vertebra
N. aortic arch

B. is correct.
The lining of the gut is endodermal in origin, but the smooth muscle of the gut forms from the splanchnic layer of the lateral plate mesoderm. Visceral peritoneum also forms from splanchnic mesoderm, but the parietal layers of the serous membranes (peritoneum, pleura, pericardium) form from the somatic layer of lateral plate mesoderm.

5.026 Which of the following is derived from the intermediate mesoderm?

A. enamel of the teeth
B. smooth muscle of the gut
C. mucous lining of the larynx
D. sympathetic chain ganglia
E. ureter
F. suprarenal medulla
G. patella
H. skeletal muscle of the upper limb
I. parietal peritoneum
J. lining of the lungs
K. spinal cord
L. parenchyma of the pancreas
M. eleventh thoracic vertebra
N. aortic arch

E. is correct.
Kidneys and ureter develop from the intermediate mesoderm. Somites and their derivatives develop from paraxial mesoderm, and lateral plate mesoderm becomes either connective tissues of the body wall and limbs (somatic layer of lateral plate mesoderm) or gut wall (splanchnic layer).

SECTION 6: PLACENTA AND FETAL MEMBRANES

6.001 The umbilical cord may loop around the fetus or become knotted, which may cause fetal distress.

A. true
B. false

A. is correct.
It is possible that the umbilical cord can loop or knot and cause fetal distress by reducing umbilical vessel flow. The umbilical cord can loop around neck or limbs, thereby making a cesarean delivery necessary.

6.002 When the amount of amniotic fluid exceeds two liters, the condition is called:

A. oligohydramnios
B. polyhydramnios or hydramnios
C. amniotitis
D. bag of waters
E. hydrogravida

B. is correct.
Polyhydramnios is a condition of excess amniotic fluid exceeding 1.5 liters. It is often caused by failure of the fetus to drink the normal amount of amniotic fluid, and may be due to anencephaly, esophageal atresia, or an upper GI tract blockage. Oligohydramnios, too little amniotic fluid, may indicate urinary problems.

6.003 The wall of the chorionic sac is composed of:

A. cytotrophoblast and syncytiotrophoblast
B. two layers of trophoblast lined by extraembryonic somatic mesoderm
C. trophoblast and exocoelomic membrane
D. extraembryonic splanchnic mesoderm & both layers of trophoblast
E. none of the above

B. is correct.
The outer layer of chorionic sac is the cytotrophoblast shell; the sac is lined with extraembryonic mesoderm of somatic type, because it does not contact the yolk sac; lining the intervillous space is syncytium. Later, the amniotic sac pushes up against and fuses to the chorionic sac, obliterating the chorionic cavity.

6.004 The most distinctive characteristic of a primary chorionic villus is its:

A. outer syncytiotrophoblastic layer
B. cytotrophoblastic shell
C. extraembryonic somatic mesodermal core
D. bushy appearance
E. cytotrophoblastic core

E. is correct.
All chorionic villi possess an outer layer of syncytiotrophoblast. The cytotrophoblast shell is a feature of the mature chorion. Extraembryonic somatic mesoderm forms the core of secondary villi, becoming tertiary with vascular development. Primary villi, at 14 days, are syncytial processes with a core of cytotrophoblast.

6.005 Chorionic villi are designated as secondary chorionic villi when they:

A. contact the decidua basalis
B. are covered by syncytiotrophoblast
C. develop a mesenchymal core
D. give rise to branch villi
E. none of the above

C. is correct.
All chorionic villi possess an outer layer of syncytiotrophoblast. The cytotrophoblast shell is a feature of the mature chorion. Extraembryonic somatic mesoderm forms the core of secondary villi, becoming tertiary with vascular development. Primary villi, at 14 days, are syncytial processes with a core of cytotrophoblast.

6.006 When chorionic villi become vascularized they are called ____ villi.

A. branch
B. stem
C. tertiary
D. anchoring
E. mature

C. is correct.
As secondary chorionic villi become vascularized, they become known as tertiary villi. Maturation of the villi involves thinning of the placental barrier, so that only a thin layer of syncytium, extracellular matrix and endothelium separates maternal and fetal blood.

6.007 The most important region of the decidua for the nourishment of the conceptus is the decidua ______.

A. frondosum
B. capsularis
C. parietalis
D. basalis
E. laeve

D. is correct.
The placenta is made of maternal tissue, the decidua basalis, and fetal tissue, the chorion frondosum or bushy/villous chorion. The smooth chorion or chorion laeve is covered by decidua capsularis, which disappears as the fetus grows and smooth chorion pushes up against the decidua parietalis.

6.008 The intervillous space contains all of the following substances EXCEPT:

A. oxygen
B. carbon dioxide
C. maternal blood cells
D. fetal blood
E. electrolytes

D. is correct.
Maternal blood cells find their way through the dark intervillous space with electrolytes, oxygen and other good things, and they carry away bad things like carbon dioxide and fetal waste products. However, fetal blood does not normally enter the intervillous space but is separated from it by the placental barrier.

6.009 Which of the following materials usually do not cross the placental membrane or barrier?

A. free fatty acids
B. steroid hormones
C. bacteria
D. vitamins
E. viruses

C. is correct.
Nutrients, gases, waste products, hormones and antibodies are items exchanged through the placental barrier. Unfortunately, some harmful things may also be transported. These include: drugs, viruses and harmful antibodies and hormones. Most bacteria are not allowed through, but syphilis Treponema may reach the fetus.

6.010 The tissue of the four-week embryo that lies in contact with the decidua basalis is:

A. cytotrophoblast shell
B. syncytiotrophoblast villi
C. chorion laeve
D. extraembryonic somatic mesoderm
E. all of the above

A. is correct.
As the chorionic villi are forming during the third week, cells of the cytotrophoblast layer form a shell around the chorion. Following this, the syncytium lines the intervillous space, primarily. Some villi attach to the cytotrophoblast shell: these are the anchoring villi.

6.011 At or near term, the intervillous space has a total volume of:

A. 150 ml
B. 400 ml
C. 500 ml
D. 1000 ml
E. 1500-2000 ml

A. is correct.
A liter of blood is a bit unbelievable. Near term, the intervillous space contains approximately 150 ml of maternal blood. Circulation is fairly rapid, and this blood is replenished three to four times per minute.

6.012 The primary source of fetal energy is:

A. the fetal intestines
B. the placenta
C. amniotic fluid
D. maternal fat

B. is correct.
The placenta is the only connection between the fetus and the world outside. Nutrients such as glucose pass through the placental membrane readily. Vitamins, water and fat soluble, cross placenta also, although the latter cross more slowly. Cholesterol and fats do not cross, but limited amounts of free fatty acids do.

6.013 The portion of the decidua which does not survive until the end of pregnancy is the:

A. capsularis
B. basalis
C. laeve
D. parietalis
E. frondosum

A. is correct.
Chorion frondosum and the decidua basalis make up the placenta. Chorion laeve, or smooth chorion, is covered by decidua capsularis. As the fetus and chorion enlarge, the chorion laeve pushes against the decidua parietalis and the capsularis disappears.

6.014 Attachment of the umbilical cord to the fetal membranes instead of to the placenta is called:

A. battledore placenta
B. Wharton's placenta
C. velamentous insertion
D. cotyledon placenta
E. eccentric insertion

C. is correct.
If umbilical cord attaches to the fetal membranes, it is called velamentous insertion, which is certainly also eccentric. If the umbilical cord inserts onto the margin of placenta, it is called a battledore placenta because it resembles a racquet. Wharton's jelly is mucopolysaccharide material surrounding the umbilical vessels.

6.015 Amniotic fluid IS NOT concerned with:

A. regulation of fetal temperature
B. exchange of fetal wastes
C. protection of the conceptus
D. early nutrition of the embryo

D. is correct.
Amniotic fluid arises from the amniotic membrane, diffusion from the decidua, and from fetal urine. It helps in maintaining constant fetal body temperature, and it provides protection for the fetus and a non-restrictive environment in which to grow and move. Exchange of wastes happens, but is not an essential feature.

6.016 Which of the following is NOT true concerning decidua basalis:

A. lies between the villous chorion and the myometrium
B. forms the "roof" of the placenta
C. supplies blood to the intervillous spaces
D. is partially composed of fetal tissues

D. is correct.
All decidual tissues are maternal tissues only. Decidua basalis is the roof of the placenta, especially if you consider the typical posterior implantation site and the normal anteverted position of the uterus. Spiral vessels from the basalis enter the intervillous space. Basalis lies between bushy chorion and myometrium.

6.017 Mechanisms involved in placental transfer of material include:

A. facilitated diffusion
B. pinocytosis
C. active transport
D. simple diffusion
E. all of the above are correct

E. is correct.
All of these mechanisms are involved in the transport of material across the placental membrane or barrier.

6.018 Which of the following is NOT true concerning the umbilical cord?

A. it usually attaches near the center of the placenta
B. it may not be attached to the placenta
C. it normally contains two arteries and one vein
D. it may form a knot that can cause fetal distress
E. it contains cardiac jelly

E. is correct.
Typically, attachment of the cord is near the center of the placenta, although it may occur marginally, called battledore placenta, or into fetal membranes, called velamentous insertion. Wharton's jelly surrounds two umbilical arteries and one vein, normally. Kinks or knots in the cord can cause fetal distress or death.

6.019 The chorionic sac surrounds the embryo, amniotic sac and yolk sac.

A. true
B. false

A. is correct.
During the embryonic period, the chorionic cavity and sac surrounds the embryo, yolk sac and amniotic sac. Later, however, the growth of the fetus and amniotic sac obliterates the chorionic cavity, and the amnion and chorion fuse to form the amniochorionic membrane.

6.020 Which of the following is NOT a component of the mature placental barrier?

A. the endothelial lining of fetal capillaries
B. the cytotrophoblast
C. the syncytiotrophoblast
D. the basement membrane of fetal capillaries
E. all of the above are part of the mature placental barrier

B. is correct.
In the last half of pregnancy, the cytotrophoblast & extraembryonic mesoderm layers are lost from the placental barrier, leaving only syncytium, capillary basement membrane and capillary endothelium between maternal and fetal circulations.

6.021 Which is NOT true concerning the human placenta:

A. is divided into a number of cup-like compartments by incomplete septae of maternal tissue
B. has an intervillous space filled with maternal blood and lined by syncytiotrophoblast
C. has chorionic villi as functional units
D. is anchored to maternal tissue by columns of syncytiotrophoblast

D. is correct.
The chorionic villi are the functional units of the placenta. The villi protrude into the intervillous spaces that are filled with maternal blood. Also penetrating the intervillous spaces are incomplete septae formed from the decidua basalis. These incomplete septae partially divide the placenta into cotyledons.

6.022 In placenta praevia, the placenta may detach and cause severe bleeding and fetal anoxia during delivery.

A. true
B. false

A. is correct.
When the placenta overbridges the internal os of the uterus, it is called placenta praevia. This can cause severe bleeding during the later stages of pregnancy and delivery.

6.023 The human placenta:

A. has a maternal component formed by the decidua capsularis
B. shows no changes with age
C. retains the cytotrophoblast layer of the placental barrier throughout gestation
D. has chorionic villi as the structural and functional unit

D. is correct.
The placenta is formed by the interconnection of the fetal chorion frondosum and the maternal decidua basalis. As the fetus grows, so does the placenta, which also loses the cytotrophoblast layer of the placental barrier. It has the chorionic villi as its fundamental units.

6.024 The placental intervillous space:

A. is divided into compartments by the placental septa
B. is a continuous space throughout the placenta
C. is lined by syncytiotrophoblast
D. contains circulating maternal blood
E. all of the above are correct

E. is correct.
The intervillous space contains maternal blood and is completely lined by syncytiotrophoblast. It is divided into cotyledons by septae from the decidua, but because these septae are incomplete, there remains communication between the compartments.

6.025 Under normal conditions, the placenta acts as a barrier against:

A. transfer of drugs and their metabolites
B. transfer of all infectious agents
C. transfer of nutrients
D. mixing of maternal and fetal blood
E. transfer of hormones

D. is correct.
The placenta does not provide a strong barrier against drugs, as most will pass through it. There are also many infectious agents that can cross the placenta and cause severe malformations. The placenta is obviously not a barrier to nutrients, but does prevent mixing of maternal and fetal blood.

6.026 Human chorionic gonadotropin (HCG) is produced by the:

A. syncytiotrophoblast
B. anterior pituitary gland
C. theca folliculi
D. corpus luteum of pregnancy
E. embryoblast

A. is correct.
It is the syncytiotrophoblast that does the job of making HCG. HCG maintains the corpus luteum and stimulates it to release both estrogen and progesterone, which inhibit menstruation and allow the pregnancy to continue. HCG can also be detected in the urine of a pregnant woman, an early indication of pregnancy.

6.027 Which of the following materials usually cross the placental membrane?

A. free fatty acids
B. steroid hormones
C. drugs and chemicals with a molecular weight of less than 500
D. vitamins
E. all of the above

E. is correct.
All of the mentioned items can cross the placenta. The placenta also transmits many viral agents, maternal antibodies or IgGs and nutrients such as amino acids and carbohydrates.

6.028 Which structure is responsible for transport of nutrients to the fetus?

A. cytotrophoblastic shell
B. trophoblast
C. decidua basalis
D. cotyledon
E. spiral artery
F. intervillous space
G. tertiary villus
H. umbilical artery
I. umbilical vein
J. syncytial knots
K. vitelline duct
L. chorion frondosum
M. amnion

I. is correct.
The paired umbilical arteries carry blood from the fetus to the placenta, to exchange wastes for nutrients and oxygen. Blood returns to the fetus in the umbilical vein, carrying nutrients and oxygen obtained from maternal blood bathing the chorionic villi.

6.029 Which structure is found in the umbilical cord, but is not part of the fetal circulatory system?

A. cytotrophoblastic shell
B. trophoblast
C. decidua basalis
D. cotyledon
E. spiral artery
F. intervillous space
G. tertiary villus
H. umbilical artery
I. umbilical vein
J. syncytial knots
K. vitelline duct
L. chorion frondosum
M. amnion

K. is correct.
The vitelline duct or yolk sac stalk connects the fetal gut with the yolk sac. As the fetus grows, the yolk sac and vitelline duct regress and disappear. However, remnants of the vitelline duct may persist within the fetus, and manifest as vitelline duct cyst, fistula, or Meckel's diverticulum.

6.030 Which of the following structures should normally be found as a pair?

A. cytotrophoblastic shell
B. trophoblast
C. decidua basalis
D. cotyledon
E. spiral artery
F. intervillous space
G. tertiary villus
H. umbilical artery
I. umbilical vein
J. syncytial knot
K. vitelline duct
L. chorion frondosum
M. amnion

H. is correct.
Two umbilical arteries an a single umbilical vein are normal. At birth, a section of the umbilical cord is taken to analyze for SUA or singe umbilical artery, which has a high correlation with birth defects.

SECTION 7: CONGENITAL MALFORMATIONS

7.001 Which of the following is true concerning fetal testing?

A. amniocentesis may be done after 2 months
B. ultrasonography is routinely performed throughout the second and third trimesters
C. alpa-fetoprotein levels in maternal blood may be suppressed in cases of fetal neural tube defects
D. chorionic villi samples and amniotic cell cultures can indicate neural tube defects

B. is correct.
Withdrawal and analysis of the amniotic fluid, or amniocentesis, may be performed at 14 weeks. Elevated alpha-fetoprotein levels in this fluid or maternal blood may indicate neural tube defects. It has become routine to perform ultrasonography during pregnancy. Samples of chorionic villi can indicate chromosomal abnormalities.

7.002 Cri du chat is a malformation which:

A. is the result of partial deletion of chromosome 5
B. results from breaking chromosome 5
C. is characterized by mental retardation, with possible cardiac defects and microcephaly
D. is named because of the high, cat-like cry of the infant
E. all of the above are correct

E. is correct.
Cri du chat syndrome results from breakage and loss of the terminal portion of chromosome 5. The syndrome is characterized by severe mental retardation, cardiac defects and microcephaly. The syndrome is named because of the cat-like cry of the affected infant.

7.003 Sex chromosome abnormalities include:

A. XO - Turner's syndrome
B. XXY - Klinefelter's syndrome
C. XYY - supermale syndrome
D. XXX - triple X syndrome
E. all of the above are correct

E. is correct.
These chromosome numerical abnormalities result from nondisjunction. Turner's shows webbed neck, barrel chest & mental retardation. Klinefelter's is anatomically male with female secondary sex traits. Supermale may have slight retardation & possibly more aggression. Triple X have slight retardation & child-like appearance.

7.004 Trisomy of somatic chromosomes is often associated with mental retardation. Which one of the following is NOT a somatic trisomy:

A. trisomy 21 - Down's syndrome
B. trisomy 13 syndrome
C. trisomy 18 syndrome
D. trisomy 24 syndrome

D. is correct.
Trisomies result from nondisjunction of homologous chromosomes. Down's syndrome is more common in advanced maternal age. Trisomy 18 shows retardation, heart defects & flexed fingers. Trisomy 13 is characterized by retardation & bilateral cleft lip/palate. Humans only have 23 pairs of chromosomes, and the 23rd is sex, not somatic.

7.005 A drug prescribed for acne that may cause serious birth defects is:

A. diethylstilbesterol
B. thalidomide
C. isotretinoin
D. organic mercury
E. progestin

C. is correct.
Isotretinoin, a vitamin A analogue, is given orally for treatment of acne, and is linked to serious facial & other defects. Thalidomide was a sedative which caused severe limb reduction deformities. DES may increase cancer risk in offspring. Mercury contaminated food has caused neurological problems. Progestins prevent ovulation.

7.006 Concerning birth defects:
- A. Chromosomal aberrations are responsible for 85% of congenital malformations.
- B. A single teratogen may produce a variety of malformations.
- C. Most malformations are induced prior to implantation.
- D. The incidence of specific malformations is the same worldwide.
- E. Malformations cannot be detected in utero.

B. is correct.
Congenital malformations of many types can be produced by a single teratogen, often depending on the stage of development of the fetus when the insult occurred. Rubella virus, for example, may cause eye, ear, cardiac, dental, or CNS defects, depending on the time of infection.

7.007 Concerning the induction of birth defects:
- A. Most malformations probably result from interactions between genetic and environmental factors.
- B. The period of organogenesis is highly susceptible to teratogenesis.
- C. The teratogenic effect depends on the concentration of the teratogen and duration of exposure.
- D. Results of altered development are death, malformation, growth retardation & functional deficit.
- E. all of the above are correct

E. is correct.
Most malformations occur while the organs are forming and are the result of interactions between genetic and environmental factors. Effect of a teratogen also depends on quantities and how long the embryo is exposed. As a result, you can have death, malformation, growth retardation, or functional deficit.

7.008 Congenital malformations may be caused by:
- A. environmental factors
- B. infectious agents
- C. radiation
- D. chromosomal anomalies
- E. all of the above are correct

E. is correct.
Congenital malformations may be caused by environmental factors, infectious agents, chemical agents, radiation, hormones, chromosomal anomalies, or combinations of the above.

7.009 Drugs and chemicals appear to account for 1% of congenital malformations.
- A. true
- B. false

A. is correct.
Although it is difficult to establish clear cause and effect with drugs and chemicals because they are so universally present, it is estimated that they cause about 1% of congenital malformations.

7.010 The fetal period appears to be the most susceptible to the action of teratogens.
- A. true
- B. false

B. is correct.
The most susceptible period to teratogenesis is the embryonic period, in which organogenesis is taking place. However, fetal growth and brain maturation can be hindered by chronic exposure to agents during the fetal period. Common drug activities like smoking and alcohol can retard fetal growth.

7.011 Alcohol is a human teratogen.
- A. true
- B. false

A. is correct.
Fetal alcohol syndrome is associated with maternal alcohol consumption and includes defects such as craniofacial abnormalities, limb deformities, cardiovascular defects, mental retardation and growth retardation.

7.012 Trisomy 21 (Down's syndrome) is an autosomal defect that is most likely due to a single gene mutation.

A. true
B. false

B. is correct.
Trisomy is the result of nondisjunction during oogenesis, causing an extra chromosome to be incorporated into the zygote. This is not a single gene mutation.

7.013 Which of the following factors affect the action of a teratogenic agent?

A. duration of exposure to the agent
B. genotype of the embryo
C. dose of the agent
D. stage of development at time of exposure
E. all of the above are correct

E. is correct.
The actual teratogenic effect depends on many things. Among them are when exposure occurred, the dose of the teratogen, and how long the embryo was exposed. It also depends upon the interaction between the teratogen and the genetic composition of the embryo.

7.014 No animal test is likely to be an absolute predictor of teratogenic action in pregnant women because:

A. lab animals are not susceptible to the same teratogens as humans
B. the duration of pregnancy in lab animals is too short to allow malformations to be induced
C. lab animals are polytocous meaning multiple young; women usually a single birth, known as monotocous
D. the pharmacokinetics of teratogens may differ between humans and animals

D. is correct.
Animal tests are not precise indicators of teratogenicity because uptake, metabolism, distribution and elimination of a teratogen may differ radically between species. In this sense, the pharmacokinetics are very different. Polytocous & monotocous mean multiple and single birth, and that would not affect teratogenic action.

7.015 Known human teratogens include:

A. alcohol
B. x-radiation
C. maternal diabetes
D. rubella virus
E. all of the above are correct

E. is correct.
Alcohol exposure can cause fetal alcohol syndrome, characterized by craniofacial, limb & heart defects & mental retardation. Rubella can cause heart & head defects, while x-rays cause diverse defects. Maternal diabetes increases the risk of malformations, including hindlimb & heart defects, as well as a high birth weight.

7.016 Chromosomal aberrations:

A. may cause malformations because of numerical excess or deficiency
B. may occur in a high percentage of spontaneous abortuses
C. may cause malformations because of structural abnormalities
D. include trisomies of sex chromosomes
E. all of the above are correct

E. is correct.
Chromosomal aberrations may involve an abnormal number of chromosomes (including sex chromosomes), breaks in chromosomes, or single gene mutations. They may cause a great majority of spontaneous abortions.

7.017 Which of the following anomalies is more common in live-born males than in live-born females?

A. pyloric stenosis
B. dislocated hip
C. birthmarks
D. brain defects
E. all of the above

A. is correct.
Pyloric stenosis, in which the pyloric lumen is severely narrowed and food passage is obstructed, is more common in live-born males than in live-born females.

7.018 In which of the following syndromes is late maternal age believed to be a major factor?

A. Cri du Chat syndrome
B. Turner's syndrome
C. Down's syndrome
D. Edwards' syndrome
E. Klinefelter's syndrome

C. is correct.
It is Down's syndrome that is particularly associated with late maternal age. It is speculated that because the primary oocytes of an older woman have spent so much time in "limbo" during the first meiotic division there is more likelihood of the occurrence of a nondisjunction.

7.019 All the following microorganisms are known to cause major congenital malformations EXCEPT:

A. treponema pallidum (Syphilis)
B. varicella (Chicken pox)
C. cytomegalovirus (CMV)
D. toxoplasma gondii
E. rubella virus

B. is correct.
Syphilis, CMV, toxoplasma and rubella can all produce severe malformations in the developing fetus. Chicken pox, on the other hand, is not as closely linked to congenital malformations, although it may cause abnormal development in some cases.

SECTION 8: MUSCLES, SKELETON AND SKIN

8.001 Hair arises from which type of tissue?

A. ectoderm
B. mesoderm
C. epidermis
D. dermis
E. more than one of the above

E. is correct.
The epidermis arises from ectoderm, and mesoderm gives rise to the dermis of the skin. Hair follicles are hybrid structures, but are primarily derived from the epidermis layer of the skin. Lanugo hair covers the fetus, and may serve to anchor the vernix caseosa to the fetal skin. Vernix may function to lubricate & protect skin.

8.002 Congenital absence of hair is called:

A. hypertrichosis
B. anonychia
C. athelia or amastia
D. pili torti
E. atrichia or alopecia

E. is correct.
Congenital alopecia or atrichia is absence of hair, and is often associated with abnormalities of other ectodermal derivatives, such as teeth or nails. Hypertrichosis is excess hair, which may be regional. Athelia is nipple absence, while amastia is absence of a breast. Anonychia is nail absence. Pili torti is bent hair.

8.003 The breast develops along the mammary line/ridge, or the milk line. Which of the following is a possible site for accessory nipples or breasts?

A. cubital fossa or anterior elbow
B. popliteal fossa or behind the knee
C. groin
D. lower lateral neck above clavicle
E. mid-axillary line at the 5th intercostal space

C. is correct.
The milk line extends from the axilla or arm pit, through the nipple and into the groin or medial thigh. Accessory nipples (polythelia) or accessory breasts (polymastia) may occur anywhere along these bilateral lines. Breasts develop from the thickened epidermis of the mammary ridge as branching ectodermal ingrowths.

8.004 Which of the following is NOT considered a "birthmark"?

A. angioma
B. hemangioma
C. port wine stain
D. ichthyosis

D. is correct.
Most birthmarks are angiomas, vascular malformations beneath the skin, although some birthmarks are aggregations of melanocytes. A port wine stain, displayed by Russian ex-President Gorbachev, is a type of angioma called a hemangioma. Ichthyosis is a skin defect involving excess keratinization, resulting in scaling.

8.005 Failure of the brain to grow may result in:

A. plagiocephaly
B. craniostenosis
C. acrocephaly
D. scaphocephaly
E. microcephaly

E. is correct.
If the brain does not grow, neither will the skull. This results in microcephaly. Premature closure of cranial sutures is called craniostenosis. Early sagittal suture fusion causes scaphocephaly or a long skull. Early coronal fusion causes acrocephaly or tower skull. Asymmetric fusions produce plagiocephaly.

8.006 Which of the following is NOT true concerning skeletal development?

A. Membrane bones include the clavicle and the bones of the cranial vault and face.
B. During membrane bone formation, no cartilaginous model is formed.
C. Endochondral bone formation involves calcification of cartilage, which is later replaced by true bone.
D. Membrane bone lacks periosteum.

D. is correct.
A bonc is a living organ, and all bone possesses a periosteal cover. Periosteum is one of the tissues which enables bones to remodel according the functional stresses. Membrane bone forms within fibrous connective tissue; no cartilaginous anlage or model forms as in endochondral bone formation.

8.007 Lobster claw deformity is characterized by:

A. ectrodactyly
B. brachydactyly
C. syndactyly
D. polydactyly
E. more than one of the above

E. is correct.
Lobster claw deformity involves loss of the middle digit and fusion of the two remaining pairs of digits, or syndactyly. Loss of digits is called ectrodactyly; brachydactyly is short digits; polydactyly is supernumerary digits. Amelia is absent limb, sympodia is fusion of the lower limbs.

8.008 Klippel-Feil syndrome is characterized by:

A. short neck due to small cervical vertebrae
B. torticollis
C. high forehead
D. restricted movements of the neck

D. is correct.
Klippel-Feil syndrome involves reduction and fusions of cervical vertebrae, reducing neck mobility. Low hairline may also be seen. Torticollis or wry-neck results from damage to sternocleidomastoid muscle of the neck on one side, usually at delivery. The head is tilted and twisted.

8.009 Somitomeres, paraxial mesoderm cranial to the somites, give rise to much of the skeletal muscle in the head EXCEPT:

A. extrinsic muscles of the eye
B. temporalis
C. tongue muscles
D. muscles of facial expression
E. muscles of mastication

C. is correct.
Somitomeres provide myotomal tissue for skeletal muscle development to the head. Muscles of somitomere origin include the extrinsic eye muscles, the muscles of facial expression, and the muscles of mastication, of which temporalis is one. Tongue muscles and the muscles of the larynx are from somitic myotomes.

8.010 The sphenoid bone is derived from which portion of the embryonic skull?

A. cartilaginous neurocranium
B. membranous neurocranium
C. cartilaginous viscerocranium
D. membranous viscerocranium
E. branchial cartilage

A. is correct.
The skull consists of two parts, the neurocranium, which forms the vault protecting the brain, and the viscerocranium, which forms the bones of the face. The base of the skull, of which sphenoid is part, develops from the cartilaginous neurocranium because it forms by endochondral ossification. Skull vault is membranous.

8.011 Which of the following is NOT true with respect to the development and growth of bones:

A. Primary centers of ossification appear before the end of the third month of development.
B. Almost all secondary ossification centers appear after birth.
C. Longitudinal growth of a long bone occurs in the areas of the epiphyseal plates.
D. Membrane bones can be recognized by their typical histological structure.

D. is correct.
Primary ossification centers appear in the shafts of long bones by the twelfth week. Secondary centers appear in the ends or epiphyses postnatally, and growth in length of a long bone occurs at the epiphyseal cartilage plate separating diaphysis & epiphysis. After development, membrane bone is not distinctive histologically.

8.012 Achondroplasia is characterized by all of the following EXCEPT:

A. inferior sexual development
B. short limbs
C. average intelligence
D. broad, flat face
E. undershot jaw

A. is correct.
Achondroplasia is a disturbance of endochondral ossification during gestation. Therefore, it affects endochondral bones and would not affect intelligence or sexual development.

8.013 Digits which are abnormally short are called:

A. syndactyly
B. polydactyly
C. dichuris
D. amelus
E. none of the above

E. is correct.
Brachydactyly is the term for shortness of the digits. It is usually inherited as a dominant trait and is often associated with short stature.

8.014 The nerve supply to a muscle can be used as an indicator of:

A. the time of differentiation of a particular muscle
B. the primary germ layer from which a given muscle arose
C. the time of myofibril formation in the muscle
D. the level of origin and path of migration of the muscle

D. is correct.
The nerve supply says nothing about the time sequence of muscular development, and we all know that muscle is of mesodermal origin, regardless of its innervation. However, the nerve supply of a muscle does indicate its level of origin and path of migration.

8.015 The notochord is replaced by the:

A. ependyma
B. vertebral column
C. spinal canal
D. dorsal roots
E. spinal cord

B. is correct.
The notochord is the forerunner of the vertebral column. As it is replaced by the vertebral column, it degenerates. All that remains of the notochord in the adult is the nucleus pulposus in the intervertebral discs, surrounded by the sclerotome-derived annulus fibrosus.

SECTION 9: BODY CAVITIES AND MEMBRANES

9.001 The intraembryonic coelom located cranial to the oropharyngeal membrane becomes the:

A. oral cavity
B. cranial foregut
C. stomodeum
D. pericardial cavity
E. nasal cavity

D. is correct.
The cardiogenic region lies cranial to the prochordal plate and its descendant, the oropharyngeal membrane. The heart tubes form on the endoderm side of intraembryonic coelom in the cardiogenic region. Following the head and lateral body folding, heart and its portion of intraembryonic coelom called pericardial cavity lie in the chest.

9.002 In the five-week embryo, the ventral mesentery of the primitive gut disappears, except where it is attached to the:

A. cranial region of the foregut
B. embryonic part of the yolk sac
C. caudal region of the hindgut
D. caudal region of the foregut
E. cranial region of the midgut

D. is correct.
The only portion of the ventral mesentery to remain is the part attaching to the caudal foregut. This is essentially the ventral mesogastrium, although it includes an attachment to the first part of the duodenum. This latter part becomes hepatoduodenal ligament. Liver & gall bladder develop in the ventral mesentery.

9.003 The intraembryonic coelom first appears during the _____ week.

A. second
B. third
C. fourth
D. fifth
E. sixth

B. is correct.
During the third week, spaces appear within the embryonic mesoderm laterally. These spaces coalesce to form a horseshoe-shaped cavity at the cranial end of the embryo called the intraembryonic coelom. This coelom is continuous with the extraembryonic coelom laterally. The coelom divides mesoderm into somatic & splanchnic layers.

9.004 Most myoblasts or muscle-forming cells of the diaphragm arise from mesenchymal cells originating in:

A. septum transversum
B. cervical somites
C. thoracic body wall
D. splanchnic mesoderm
E. neural crest

B. is correct.
All skeletal muscle originates from somitic myotomes, and the muscle of the diaphragm is skeletal muscle. The cervical myotome cells enter the developing diaphragm during its descent to its final location. Because nerves always follow muscle regardless of its migration, the phrenic nerves, C3-5, innervate the diaphragm.

9.005 Which of the following is NOT true concerning development of the diaphragm?

A. The phrenic nerves pass through the pleuropericardial membranes to reach the diaphragm.
B. The sole motor nerves to the diaphragm arise from spinal cord segments at cervical levels three, four and five.
C. The periphery of the diaphragm is supplied by sensory branches of the intercostal nerves.
D. Phrenic nerves form during the 8th week as septum transversum lies at the level of the cervical somites.

D. is correct.
Phrenic nerves, from C3-5, reach the diaphragm slightly later than 4th week, when septum transversum lies at cervical levels. Phrenic nerves are the sole motor nerves to the diaphragm, but intercostal branches innervate it peripherally. Phrenic nerves pass through the pleuropericardial membranes, later fibrous pericardium.

9.006 Which of the following is true concerning congenital diaphragmatic hernia through a posterolateral defect?

A. It is the most common type of diaphragmatic hernia.
B. Stomach, intestines and part of liver may herniate into the thoracic cavity.
C. It occurs more often on the left side.
D. The lungs may be compressed and hypoplastic.
E. all of the above are correct

E. is correct.
Posterolateral diaphragmatic hernia involves failure of closure of the pleuroperitoneal canals. It usually occurs on the left, and parts of stomach, spleen, intestine and liver may pass up into the chest, compressing lungs. Diaphragmatic hernia is a fairly common malformation, and a posterolateral defect is the most common type.

9.007 The pleuropericardial membranes give rise to the fibrous pericardium of the adult. In the embryo, these membranes contain:

A. lung buds
B. cardinal veins
C. dorsal aortae
D. phrenic nerves
E. more than one of the above

E. is correct.
Initially, the pleuropericardial folds seem to be pushed out by the common cardinal veins. They contain the phrenic nerves at their bases. The folds merge behind the heart. Lung buds are always behind or below the pleuropericardial folds or membranes. Dorsal aorta is also behind, on the posterior body wall.

9.008 Which of the following gives rise to pleura?

A. ectoderm
B. splanchnic mesoderm
C. endoderm
D. somatic mesoderm
E. more than one of the above

E. is correct.
Mesoderm lines the intraembryonic coelom, and is divided by the coelom into somatic, associated with body wall, and splanchnic, associated with gut, layers. The somatic mesoderm lining becomes the parietal layers of pleura, serous pericardium & peritoneum. Visceral serous membranes come from splanchnic mesoderm.

9.009 Which of the following does NOT contribute to the diaphragm:

A. body wall musculature
B. pleuroperitoneal membranes
C. septum transversum
D. ventral mesentery

D. is correct.
The first three items mentioned are components of the diaphragm. A defect in the pleuroperitoneal membrane can result in a diaphragmatic hernia, in which abdominal contents herniate into the thoracic cavity, usually on the left side. This can interfere with the development of the lung, making it hypoplastic.

9.010 Growth of the pleuropericardial membranes is due to:

A. descent of the heart
B. expansion of pleural cavities
C. growth of common cardinal veins ventrocranially
D. expansion of the pericardial cavity
E. more than one of the above

E. is correct.
The pleuropericardial membranes develop from the pleuropericardial folds and contain the phrenic nerves and common cardinal veins. Via descent of the heart and the ventrocranial growth of the common cardinal veins, these membranes are brought into apposition, ultimately forming the fibrous pericardium.

9.011 The intraembryonic coelom:
A. gives rise to pleural, pericardial and peritoneal cavities
B. has a communication with the amniotic cavity
C. splits the lateral plate mesoderm
D. is continuous with the yolk sac
E. more than one of the above

E. is correct.
The lateral plate mesoderm splits into somatic mesoderm, which lines the body wall, and splanchnic mesoderm, which lines the yolk sac. The area between these layers is the intraembryonic coelom, the progenitor of the pleural, pericardial and peritoneal cavities. In early development, it communicates with chorionic cavity.

9.012 The embryonic mesogastrium NEVER contains:
A. dorsal pancreas
B. spleen
C. mesenchyme
D. superior mesenteric artery

D. is correct.
The dorsal pancreas, spleen and mesenchyme are all contained, at one time or another, within the mesogastrium. With rotation of the stomach, however, the pancreas ultimately winds up in a retroperitoneal position. The superior mesenteric artery is the midgut artery and is therefore not in the mesogastrium.

9.013 The derivatives of the embryonic ventral mesentery include the following structures EXCEPT:
A. hepatoduodenal ligament
B. hepatogastric ligament
C. falciform ligament
D. ligamentum teres hepatis
E. lesser omentum

D. is correct.
The ligamentum teres hepatis is a remnant of the fetal umbilical vein. Although it is contained within the ventral mesentery, it is not a derivative of it.

9.014 Which of the following organs is NOT normally retroperitoneal:
A. suprarenal gland
B. pancreas
C. descending colon
D. sigmoid colon

D. is correct.
The suprarenal or adrenal glands and kidneys develop retroperitoneally. Four gut structures, the pancreas, duodenum, ascending & descending colon, develop intraperitoneally, but are pushed against the posterior body wall during gut rotation. These four structures fuse there, and are therefore called secondarily retroperitoneal.

9.015 The following peritoneal ligaments are derived wholly or in part from the embryonic dorsal mesogastrium EXCEPT:
A. hepatogastric ligament
B. splenorenal or lienorenal ligament
C. gastrosplenic or gastrolienal ligament
D. gastrocolic ligament
E. transverse mesocolon

A. is correct.
Splenorenal, gastrosplenic and gastrocolic ligaments are derived from the dorsal mesogastrium, while transverse mesocolon fuses with dorsal mesogastrium. The hepatogastric ligament, on the other hand, is derived from the ventral mesentery.

9.016 Which of the following contribute to the formation of the diaphragm?
A. septum transversum
B. mesenchyme of the costal body walls
C. both
D. neither

C. is correct.
The diaphragm is formed by: septum transversum, forming the central tendon portion; the pleuroperitoneal membranes; mesenchyme from the lateral and dorsal body walls, giving rise to the musculature of the diaphragm; and the esophageal mesentery, which gives rise to the crura of the diaphragm.

9.017 The coelom originally located cranial to the prochordal plate becomes the:

A. mouth cavity
B. stomodeum
C. pericardial cavity
D. pharyngeal cavity
E. pleural cavity

C. is correct.
Remember that early in development, the heart begins to develop beneath the intraembryonic coelom cranial to prochordal plate. The intraembryonic coelom is later subdivided into a single pericardial, paired pleural and a single peritoneal cavities. Folding of the embryo brings heart & pericardial cavity into the chest.

9.018 After folding of the head region, the structure lying just caudal to the pericardial cavity is the:

A. developing heart
B. connecting stalk
C. primitive streak
D. liver
E. septum transversum

E. is correct.
The septum transversum is the diaphragm's earliest progenitor. After folding of the head region brings the heart and its coelom region ventrally, the septum transversum is the structure that lies immediately caudal to it. Liver is not a bad guess, but remember that the diaphragm lies between it and the thorax in the adult.

9.019 Which structure develops, in part, within the septum transversum?

A. lungs
B. small intestine
C. larynx
D. esophagus
E. heart
F. stomach
G. parietal pleura
H. visceral pleura
I. liver
J. pancreas
K. ascending colon
L. transverse colon

I. is correct.
The hepatic diverticulum grows from the caudal foregut into the ventral mesentery and the septum transversum.

9.020 Which structure develops dorsal to the intraembryonic coelom in the region cranial to the prochordal plate/oropharyngeal membrane?

A. lung
B. small intestine
C. larynx
D. esophagus
E. heart
F. stomach
G. parietal pleura
H. visceral pleura
I. liver
J. pancreas
K. ascending colon
L. transverse colon

E. is correct.
The heart tubes develop dorsal to the intraembryonic coelom in the cardiogenic region at the cranial end of the embryo.

9.021 Which structure develops from the somatic layer of lateral plate mesoderm?

A. lung
B. small intestine
C. larynx
D. esophagus
E. heart
F. stomach
G. parietal pleura
H. visceral pleura
I. liver
J. pancreas
K. ascending colon
L. transverse colon

G. is correct.

The cell layer lining the intraembryonic coelom develops into the serous membranes of the three body cavities: pleura, pericardium and peritoneum. The inner lining of the somatic layer of the lateral plate mesoderm becomes the parietal layer of these serous membranes, while the outer lining of the splanchnic layer of the lateral plate becomes the visceral pleura-pericardium-peritoneum, lining the organs in these body cavities.

SECTION 10: CRANIOFACIAL REGION

10.001 Which elements are derived from neural crest?

A. head mesenchyme
B. hyoid bone
C. C-cells or parafollicular cells of the thyroid
D. thyroid cartilage
E. all of the above are correct

E. is correct.
Neural crest cells give rise to many mesenchymal structures of the pharyngeal arches, including all of those mentioned. Since neural crest is ectodermal in origin, this mesenchyme is referred to as ectomesenchyme.

10.002 The laryngeal cartilages develop from branchial arches IV and VI.

A. true
B. false

A. is correct.
Laryngeal cartilages arise from arches IV&VI. The muscles of arches IV & VI are the laryngeal muscles, pharyngeal muscles (except for stylopharyngeus) and cricothyroideus and levator veli palatini. The nerve of the 4th & 6th arches is vagus via its superior & recurrent laryngeal branches.

10.003 The parathyroid glands are derivatives of pharyngeal pouches III and IV.

A. true
B. false

A. is correct.
The thymus and inferior parathyroid arise from the 3rd pouch, while superior parathyroid arises from the 4th pouch, close to the 5th pouch derivative, the ultimobranchial body. Descent of the thymus into the chest carries parathyroid III inferior to parathyroid IV. Although variable in location, both are often found behind thyroid.

10.004 The hypobranchial eminence contributes to formation of:

A. anterior portion of the tongue
B. posterior portion of the tongue
C. musculature of the tongue
D. epiglottis
E. palatine tonsil

B. is correct.
Hypobranchial eminence forms the posterior third of the tongue. It is served by the nerve of the 3rd branchial arch, glossopharyngeal. Tongue musculature arises from occipital somites and is innervated by CN XII, hypoglossal. Epiglottis arises as an epiglottic swelling on the 4th arch. Palatine tonsil is from the 2nd pouch.

10.005 The fact that general and special sensory information from the posterior part of the tongue is carried by glossopharyngeal nerve indicates that this part of tongue is from branchial arch ____.

A. I
B. II
C. III
D. IV
E. VI

C. is correct.
Hypobranchial eminence forms the posterior third of the tongue. It is served by the nerve of the 3rd branchial arch, glossopharyngeal, or cranial nerve IX. Glossopharyngeal carries general sense and the special sense of taste from this part of the tongue. In anterior tongue, trigeminal does general and facial does special sense.

10.006 Myoblasts from the occipital myotomes are believed to give rise to the muscles of the:

A. eye
B. face
C. ear
D. jaw, for mastication
E. tongue

E. is correct.
Most of the muscles of the head arise from the somitomeres located cranial to the occipital somites. Occipital myotomes supply muscle for tongue, and are innervated by cranial nerve XII, hypoglossal.

10.007 As a resident in pediatrics, you are called to see a newborn who has a unilateral cleft lip and a unilateral cleft of the primary palate. This condition is most likely the result of:

A. failure of fusion of the mandibular prominences
B. failure of fusion of the medial nasal processes
C. failure of fusion of the maxillary prominence with the medial nasal prominence
D. failure of fusion of the lateral palatine processes with the nasal septum
E. failure of fusion of the paired lateral palatine processes

C. is correct.
This type of cleft is a failure of fusion, or secondary rupture of the union, of maxillary prominence with medial nasal prominence. If the palatine shelves or processes of maxillary prominences rupture or fail to fuse, a midline defect of the secondary palate will result.

10.008 Which of the following structures is NOT part of the first branchial arch?

A. malleus
B. mandibular process
C. sphenomandibular ligament
D. stylohyoid ligament
E. maxillary process

D. is correct.
Mandibular and maxillary processes are both from first arch, as are malleus & incus bones of the ear. Sphenomandibular ligament is the remnant of the perichondrium of Meckel's cartilage, around which the mandible forms. Second arch cartilage gives rise to stapes, styloid process, stylohyoid ligament, lesser horns & upper part of hyoid.

10.009 Which of the following structures is NOT part of the 2nd branchial arch?

A. stapes
B. superior portion of body of hyoid bone
C. sphenomandibular ligament
D. stylohyoid ligament
E. lesser cornu of the hyoid bone

C. is correct.
The cartilage of the first arch gives rise to malleus, incus, spine of sphenoid & lingula of mandible. Sphenomandibular ligament is a remnant of the perichondrium of Meckel's cartilage, also from the first arch. Second arch cartilage gives rise to stapes, styloid process, stylohyoid ligament, lesser horns & upper part of hyoid.

10.010 Which structures are derived from the intermaxillary segment of the embryonic face?

A. philtrum
B. anterior portion of the palate
C. anterior portion of the upper jaws
D. upper incisor teeth
E. all of the above are correct

E. is correct.
The intermaxillary segment gives rise to the philtrum, the upper incisors, the anterior portion of the upper jaws, and the primary palate, which lies anteriorly.

10.011 The nasolacrimal groove separates the:

A. mandibular and maxillary swellings
B. lateral nasal swelling and maxillary swelling
C. medial nasal swelling and maxillary swelling
D. first and second branchial arches
E. otic and optic vesicles

B. is correct.
The nasolacrimal groove lies between the maxillary swelling or prominence and the lateral nasal swelling. This groove ultimately forms the nasolacrimal duct and lacrimal sac. In the adult, it is the passage used by tears to travel from the eye to inferior meatus of the nasal cavity, to make your nose run when you cry.

10.012 Which of the following does NOT form from the thyroglossal duct?

A. pyramidal lobe of the thyroid
B. ectopic thyroid tissue
C. thyroglossal cyst
D. branchial fistula

D. is correct.
The thyroglossal duct can lead to the formation of the pyramidal lobe of the thyroid, ectopic thyroid tissue, or a thyroglossal duct cyst. A branchial fistula is formed by the failure of the 2nd pharyngeal arch to overgrow the 3rd and 4th clefts.

10.013 The secondary palate is formed by:

A. fusion of palatal shelves
B. posterior growth of the primary palate
C. mesenchyme of the first arch
D. cell death in the region of the oropharyngeal membrane
E. more than one of the above

E. is correct.
The secondary or definitive palate is formed by the fusion of the palatal shelves. The palatal shelves are outgrowths of the maxillary prominences, which are first arch derivatives. The secondary palate fuses with the primary palate from the intermaxillary segment to form the adult hard palate.

10.014 The branchial, visceral, or pharyngeal arches are derived from:

A. ectoderm
B. endoderm
C. both
D. neither

C. is correct.
The branchial arches contain tissue from all three germ layers. They have a mesodermal core, covered externally by ectoderm and lined internally by endoderm.

10.015 Many facial malformations are believed to be due to:

A. a failure of the oral membrane to rupture
B. a failure of neural crest cells to migrate into the facial processes
C. a failure in growth of the head fold
D. an abnormal persistence of the pharyngeal clefts
E. none of the above

B. is correct.
Proper migration of neural crest cells into the face area is vitally important to facial development. Neural crest tissue will form much of the facial skeleton.

10.016 The foramen cecum of the adult tongue:

A. marks the point of embryonic evagination of the thymus gland
B. divides the tongue into two parts, an anterior one-third and a posterior two-thirds
C. marks the point of embryonic evagination of the thyroid gland
D. develops into taste buds
E. has no embryologic significance

C. is correct.
The foramen cecum on the tongue is the point from which the thyroid gland evaginated and began its journey down into the neck. It lies at the apex of the V-shaped terminal sulcus, which divides the tongue into anterior 2/3rds, from the lateral lingual swellings and tuberculum impar, and posterior 1/3rd, from the copula.

10.017 Identify the correct associations:

A. primary palate - palatine shelves of maxillary processes
B. neural crest cells - facial processes
C. nasolacrimal groove - lateral nasal process and mandibular process
D. cleft lip - medial & lateral nasal processes

B. is correct.
The primary palate arises from the intermaxillary segment. Neural crest cells are vital to the development of the facial swellings. The nasolacrimal groove separates maxillary and lateral nasal swellings. Cleft lip can result from failure of fusion between the maxillary and medial nasal prominences.

10.018 The pharyngeal arches are associated with each of the following EXCEPT :

A. cartilaginous structures
B. cranial nerves
C. venous arches
D. vascular components
E. muscular components

C. is correct.
The pharyngeal arches have their own mesodermal core, giving rise to cartilaginous & muscular components, cranial nerve components, vascular components and derivatives of neural crest cells.

10.019 Which of the following malformations is NOT found in the "first pharyngeal arch syndrome"?

A. abnormal external ear
B. abnormal middle ear
C. macrostomia
D. thyroglossal duct cyst
E. defect in lower eye lid

D. is correct.
Connective tissue of the first arch gives rise to incus and malleus of the middle ear, the premaxilla, maxilla, zygomatic, part of the temporal bone and Meckel's cartilage for mandible development. First arch syndrome can involve various components of the face and ear.

10.020 The intermaxillary segment of the embryonic face gives rise to the philtrum of the upper lip, part of the maxilla with four incisor teeth and the triangular primary palate.

A. true
B. false

A. is correct.
The intermaxillary segment gives rise to the philtrum, the upper incisors, the anterior portion of the upper jaws and the primary palate, which lies anteriorly. This is the premaxilla of other mammals.

10.021 Cleft palate results when the palatine shelves fail to fuse with the nasal septum.

A. true
B. false

B. is correct.
The elevation or horizontal remodelling of the palatine processes of the maxillary prominences bring the palatal shelves into contact with each other and with the lower margin of the nasal septum. However, clefting of the secondary palate results from nonfusion or rupture of the fusion of the palatal shelves.

10.022 A syndrome involving a lack of pharyngeal pouch III would result in a lack of the thymus gland and palatine tonsil.

A. true
B. false

B. is correct.
The 3rd pharyngeal pouch gives rise to the inferior parathyroid glands and the thymus gland. The palatine tonsil comes from the 2nd pharyngeal pouch.

10.023 Each pharyngeal arch includes:

A. derivatives of ectodermal neural crest cells
B. an aortic arch artery
C. a mesodermal core from paraxial mesoderm
D. a cranial nerve
E. all of the above

E. is correct.
The pharyngeal arches have their own mesodermal core, giving rise to cartilaginous & muscular components, cranial nerve components, vascular components and derivatives of neural crest cells, which supplement much of the connective tissue of the face.

10.024 Which of the following are associated with the 2nd pharyngeal arch?

A. the malleus bone
B. facial nerve
C. glossopharyngeal muscle
D. the lower portion of the hyoid bone
E. anterior belly of digastric

B. is correct.
The stapes, styloid process, stylohyoid ligament, lesser horn of hyoid and upper part of hyoid body all come from 2nd arch. The nerve of the 2nd arch is CN VII or facial nerve, and the muscles are stapedius, stylohyoid, posterior belly of digastric and the muscles of facial expression.

10.025 Identify the correct associations:

A. external ear abnormality - mandibular and maxillary processes
B. oblique facial cleft - frontal and maxillary processes
C. cleft lip - maxillary & medial nasal processes
D. macrostomia - mandibular and hyoid arches
E. aglossia - mandibular arch

C. is correct.
Macro- and microstomia results from too little or too much fusion between maxillary and mandibular swellings. Oblique facial cleft represents failure of maxillary & lateral nasal process fusion. External ear develops from first pharyngeal cleft region dorsally. Cleft lip is usually between maxillary & medial nasal prominences.

10.026 Which of the following are associated with the 3rd pharyngeal pouch?

A. parafollicular or calcitonin cells of the thyroid gland
B. superior parathyroid gland
C. thyroid gland
D. thymus gland

D. is correct.
The 3rd pharyngeal pouch gives rise to the inferior parathyroid glands and the thymus gland. The parafollicular cells are from the ultimobranchial body of the 5th pharyngeal pouch. Thyroid arises from the epithelium of the pharynx, via the thyroid diverticulum.

10.027 Branchial cysts or lateral cervical cysts:

A. are found along the anterior border of the sternocleidomastoid muscle
B. are formed from a rupture of the membrane between pharyngeal pouches and branchial clefts
C. are remnants of the thyroglossal duct
D. are found in front of the ear

A. is correct.
Lateral cervical cysts are remnants of the cervical sinus, which forms when the 2nd arch grows over the 3rd & 4th arches. The cysts are found along the anterior border of the sternocleidomastoid muscle, usually just below the angle of the jaw. They have nothing to do with the rupture of anything.

10.028 An absent lower jaw is called:

A. micrognathus
B. cleft lip
C. macrostomus
D. cheiloschisis
E. agnathus

E. is correct.
The total absence of a lower jaw is termed agnathus. There is a class of fishes called agnatha with no lower jaw development.

10.029 In the process of face formation or construction, the first to come into being is the:

A. orbital ridge
B. upper jaw
C. lower jaw
D. ears
E. nose

C. is correct.
This is somewhat of a judgement call, but the mandibular arch has a complete mandibular prominence across the midline before any of these other structures are formed or fused.

10.030 Auditory ossicles develop from the condensed mesenchyme of the:

A. third branchial arch
B. fourth branchial arch
C. both
D. neither

D. is correct.
The auditory ossicles form from the mesenchyme of the 1st and 2nd pharyngeal arches. Malleus & incus come from the 1st arch, while stapes arises from the 2nd arch.

10.031 The third branchial arch cartilage gives rise to the:

A. stylohyoid ligament
B. thyroid cartilage
C. styloid process
D. greater cornu of the hyoid bone
E. sphenomandibular ligament

D. is correct.
The third arch produces the lower part of the body and the greater horns of the hyoid bone, as well as the stylopharyngeus muscle. Its nerve is the glossopharyngeal nerve. The sphenomandibular ligament is from the 1st arch. The styloid process & stylohyoid ligament are from the 2nd arch. Thyroid cartilage is from 4th arch.

10.032 A small blind pit at the anterior border of the sternocleidomastoid muscle that drips mucus is likely the persistence of the embryonic opening of the:

A. first pharyngeal pouch
B. third pharyngeal pouch
C. second branchial groove
D. second branchial groove and cervical sinus
E. thyroglossal duct

D. is correct.
The question describes a lateral cervical cyst that is draining by way of a branchial fistula. This forms due to a failure of the 2nd arch to grow caudally over the third and fourth arches, and causes the persistence of the opening of the 2nd branchial groove and the cervical sinus.

10.033 Which of the following develops from the connective tissue component of the second pharyngeal arch?

A. thyroglossal duct
B. malleus
C. tympanic membrane
D. laryngeal muscles
E. mylohyoid muscle
F. palatine tonsil
G. lesser horn of hyoid bone
H. superior parathyroid gland
I. stylopharyngeus muscle
J. nasolacrimal duct
K. cricoid cartilage
L. external auditory meatus

G. is correct.
The connective tissue of the second pharyngeal arch develops into stapedius, styloid process, stylohyoid ligament, lesser horn of the hyoid, and the upper portion of the body of the hyoid bone.

10.034 Which of the following develops from the first pharyngeal cleft?

A. thyroglossal duct
B. malleus
C. tympanic membrane
D. laryngeal muscles
E. mylohyoid muscle
F. palatine tonsil
G. lesser horn of hyoid bone
H. superior parathyroid gland
I. stylopharyngeus muscle
J. nasolacrimal duct
K. cricoid cartilage
L. external auditory meatus

L. is correct.
The external auditory meatus develops from the first pharyngeal cleft. Tympanic membrane lies between first cleft and first pouch.

10.035 Which of the following develops from the third pharyngeal arch?

A. thyroglossal duct
B. malleus
C. tympanic membrane
D. laryngeal muscles
E. mylohyoid muscle
F. palatine tonsil
G. lesser horn of hyoid bone
H. superior parathyroid gland
I. stylopharyngeus muscle
J. nasolacrimal duct
K. cricoid cartilage
L. external auditory meatus

I. is correct.
The stylopharyngeus develops from the third arch, and is innervated by the third arch nerve, glossopharyngeal (CN IX). The greater horns and lower portion of the body of the hyoid bone also develops from third arch.

SECTION 11: CARDIOVASCULAR SYSTEM

11.001 The specialized group of mesenchymal cells which aggregate to form blood islands are called:

A. hemoblasts
B. angioblasts
C. fibroblasts
D. yolk sac endoderm
E. Wharton's jelly

B. is correct.
Hemoblasts is a tempting choice, but the blood cell and blood vessel precursors are called angioblasts. Angioblasts form angiogenic cell clusters, which form blood islands centrally and primitive blood vessels peripherally. Early angiogenesis occurs in chorion, yolk sac & connecting stalk, but involves only mesodermal cells.

11.002 The cardiovascular system begins to develop during the third week.

A. true
B. false

A. is correct.
The cardiovascular system is the first organ system to become functional. At the beginning of the third week, angiogenic cell clusters appear in the wall of the yolk sac, in the chorion and in connecting stalk mesoderm. The heart tubes form within a few days, and the fused heart tube begins to beat at the end of week three.

11.003 The primitive heart is partitioned into four separate chambers during the fourth week.

A. true
B. false

B. is correct.
The formation of the four heart chambers is only beginning at the end of the fourth week, and is not complete until the end of the embryonic period.

11.004 The heart is derived from:

A. splanchnic mesoderm
B. somatic mesoderm
C. septum transversum
D. intermediate mesoderm
E. paraxial mesoderm

A. is correct.
The heart tubes form within the cardiogenic region cranial to the oropharyngeal membrane and beneath the intraembryonic coelom. If it is beneath the intraembryonic coelom, then it lies toward the yolk sac and must be splanchnic mesoderm. Somatic mesoderm would be the other side, or roof, of the intraembryonic coelom.

11.005 The dorsal mesocardium:

A. disappears partially and thereby helps to form the transverse pericardial sinus
B. disappears and helps to form the oblique pericardial sinus
C. persists as the fibrous pericardium
D. persists as the endocardium
E. fuses with the dorsal mesogastrium

A. is correct.
Early in heart development, following head folding, the heart tube is suspended within the pericardial cavity by dorsal mesocardium. As the heart folds on itself so that the intake and outflow tracts come together, the dorsal mesocardium ruptures. This forms the transverse pericardial sinus behind the great arteries.

11.006 By 13-14 days of development, angiogenic cell clusters have differentiated in the:

A. extraembryonic mesoderm of the chorion
B. splanchnic mesoderm in the wall of the yolk sac
C. connecting stalk
D. cardiogenic mesoderm
E. all of the above

E. is correct.
Angiogenic cell clusters develop in all of these areas, giving rise to the cardiovascular system in the embryo. Within the embryo, the angiogenic cell clusters are found in the horse-shoe shaped region beneath the intraembryonic coelom. Cranial to the prochordal plate lies the cardiogenic region, part of this larger area.

11.007 The most superior part of the inferior vena cava is derived from:

A. left vitelline vein
B. right vitelline vein
C. right umbilical vein
D. left umbilical vein
E. sinus venosus

B. is correct.
The vitelline veins, as they pass through the developing liver, break up into hepatic sinusoids. When the left sinus horn regresses, blood is shunted from the left vitelline vein to the right, which enlarges and ultimately forms the posthepatic portion of the inferior vena cava.

11.008 The embryonic origin of the ligamentum arteriosum is from the:

A. second arch artery
B. third arch artery
C. fourth arch artery
D. fifth arch artery
E. sixth arch artery

E. is correct.
The sixth arch is the pulmonary arch, from which pulmonary arteries are derived. On the left side, this arch maintains its connection with the dorsal aorta. In the fetus, this connection is patent and is called the ductus arteriosus. Postnatally, it closes and persists as the ligamentum arteriosum.

11.009 The bulboventricular ridge of the embryonic heart:

A. persists as the membranous part of the interventricular septum
B. becomes the upper segment of the muscular interventricular septum
C. contributes to the formation of the left atrioventricular orifice
D. gives origin to the trabeculae carneae
E. disappears without a trace

E. is correct.
The bulboventricular ridge or flange initially separates the atrioventricular canal and primitive left ventricle from the bulbus cordis. However, it regresses, allowing communication between the primitive right and left ventricles. Ultimately, it vanishes.

11.010 At birth, the following changes in circulation take place EXCEPT:

A. decrease in pressure in the pleural cavities
B. closure of the ductus venosus
C. closure of the ductus arteriosus
D. closure of the foramen ovale
E. relaxation of the thoracic diaphragm

E. is correct.
At birth, the lungs fill with air, and the pressure in the pressure in the pleural cavities begins to decline. Ductus venosus becomes ligamentum venosum. The ductus arteriosus closes and becomes the ligamentum arteriosum. Also, the foramen ovale closes and becomes the fossa ovalis.

11.011 The embryonic branchial arch arteries give origin to all of the following postnatal structures EXCEPT:

A. arch of aorta
B. ligamentum arteriosum
C. pulmonary arteries
D. ascending aorta
E. common carotid arteries

D. is correct.
Aortic arch is derived from aortic sac and left fourth arch. The ligamentum arteriosum is from the distal portion of the left sixth arch, from which the pulmonary arteries also arise. Common carotids come from third arch. The ascending aorta, however, is from the truncus arteriosus.

11.012 The following are true statements with regard to the fetal circulation EXCEPT:

A. Since the fetal liver is a hemopoietic organ, it is large and well supplied with oxygenated blood.
B. Fetal brain receives relatively pure arterial blood.
C. Fetal and maternal blood vessels anastomose in the placenta.
D. In early developmental stages, one pulmonary vein buds from the left atrium of the heart.
E. Foramen primum of the interatrial septum closes after the formation of the foramen secundum.

C. is correct.
In the placenta, there is no anastomosis between the maternal and fetal vessels. Maternal blood from the spiral arteries enters the cotyledons, where it bathes the villi from the fetus. This all occurs without anastomosis.

11.013 The following features of the adult human body represent remnants of fetal circulation EXCEPT:

A. fossa ovalis of the heart
B. musculi pectinati of the atria
C. oblique vein of the left atrium
D. ligamentum arteriosum
E. ligamentum teres hepatis

B. is correct.
The pectinate muscles are merely small muscles on the inner surface of the atria. They are not remnants of the fetal circulation, as are the fossa ovalis, oblique vein, ligamentum arteriosum and ligamentum teres hepatis. Pectinate muscles are, however, remnants of the wall of the original atrium.

11.014 Each of the following statements are correctly paired EXCEPT:

A. right vitelline vein - inferior vena cava
B. left vitelline vein - liver sinusoids
C. right anterior cardinal vein - part of superior vena cava
D. right umbilical vein - definitive umbilical vein
E. left sinus horn - coronary sinus

D. is correct.
The right umbilical vein totally disappears. The definitive umbilical vein is the left one. After birth, it closes and becomes the ligamentum teres hepatis.

11.015 The blood vessels that carry relatively "pure" arterial blood during fetal development are:

A. superior vena cava
B. inferior vena cava below liver
C. pulmonary artery
D. ascending aorta

D. is correct.
The posthepatic inferior vena cava carries oxygenated blood from the ductus venosus. Upon reaching the heart, most of this blood passes through the foramen ovale to the left heart and the ascending aorta, leaving poorly oxygenated blood entering from superior vena cava to reach right ventricle and pulmonary trunk.

11.016 The Tetralogy of Fallot includes the following defects of the heart:

A. aortic stenosis
B. dextroposition of the aorta
C. left ventricular hypertrophy
D. atrial septal defect

B. is correct.
The defects in the Tetralogy of Fallot are: pulmonary stenosis, ventricular septal defect, overriding aorta and right ventricular hypertrophy. It results from abnormal conotruncal septation. Dexter, as in dextroposition, means right; sinster means left.

11.017 The changes that normally occur shortly after birth include:

A. the umbilical vein becomes the ligamentum venosum
B. blood flow in the pulmonary arteries is reversed
C. thymus gland undergoes involution
D. the umbilical arteries become medial umbilical ligaments

D. is correct.
Around the time of birth, the distal portions of the umbilical arteries become the medial umbilical ligaments. However, the umbilical vein becomes the ligamentum teres hepatis, the blood flow in the pulmonary arteries does not reverse, and the thymus does not involute until later in life.

11.018 The following embryonic structures are involved in the formation of the definitive right atrium EXCEPT:

A. primitive atrium
B. right sinus venosus
C. left sinus venosus
D. right sinus horn
E. left sinus horn

E. is correct.
The left sinus horn regresses during development to form coronary sinus. Oblique vein of left atrium, from left common cardinal, drains to it. Coronary sinus drains blood from the heart into the right atrium.

11.019 Each of the following associations is correct EXCEPT:

A. right sinus horn - coronary sinus
B. right vitelline vein - inferior vena cava
C. right posterior cardinal vein - azygos vein
D. dorsal mesocardium - transverse sinus of the pericardium
E. umbilical veins - allantois

A. is correct.
The right sinus horn contributes greatly to the right atrium, forming the smooth-walled part of it. It does not form the coronary sinus, the left sinus horn does. Right vitelline vein forms the posthepatic portion of the IVC. Dorsal mesocardium ruptures to produce the transverse pericardial sinus.

11.020 The Tetralogy of Fallot is characterized by the following features EXCEPT:

A. stenosis of the pulmonary artery
B. interventricular septal defect
C. overriding aorta
D. hypertrophy of the left ventricle

D. is correct.
The defects in the Tetralogy of Fallot are: pulmonary stenosis, ventricular septal defect, overriding aorta and right ventricular hypertrophy. It results from unequal conotruncal septation.

11.021 Each of the following normally occurs during the neonatal period EXCEPT:

A. pressure decreases in the thoracic cavity
B. pressure increases in the left atrium
C. flattening of the alveolar epithelium of the lung
D. reversal of blood flow in the inferior vena cava
E. closure of the ductus venosus

D. is correct.
There is no reason, nor should there be any reason, for blood flow in the inferior vena cava to reverse. Such an occurrence would eliminate blood return from the lower half of the body, which is not conducive to a healthy existence.

11.022 During embryonic and fetal development:

A. venous blood from the caudal half of the body is returned by the posterior cardinal veins
B. the pulmonary arteries carry essentially oxygenated blood
C. the prehepatic inferior vena cava carries essentially oxygenated blood
D. the umbilical arteries contain oxygenated blood

A. is correct.
In the embryo, blood return from the caudal half of the body is via the posterior cardinals. Later, the POSThepatic IVC carries blood from the lower body and the ductus venosus, the latter carrying umbilical venous, oxygenated blood. The pulmonary and umbilical arteries, however, carry poorly oxygenated blood.

11.023 The heart is derived from:

A. ectoderm
B. endoderm
C. both
D. neither

D. is correct.
The heart is all mesoderm, arising from the cardiogenic area. This obviously leaves room for neither ectoderm nor endoderm to sneak into the picture, although neural crest cells do form cardiac ganglia and smooth muscle in the great vessels, and play a major role in conotruncal septation.

11.024 Each of the following ligaments in the adult are derived from fetal blood vessels EXCEPT:

A. medial umbilical ligament
B. median umbilical ligament
C. round ligament of the liver (ligamentum teres hepatis)
D. ligamentum venosum
E. ligamentum arteriosum

B. is correct.
Median umbilical ligament, attaching to upper part of bladder, is a remnant of the urachus, which itself was a remnant of the allantois. The allantois was a connection between the urinary bladder and the yolk sac, not a fetal blood vessel.

11.025 Of the following, the one most closely associated with the ligamentum teres hepatis is:

A. umbilical vein
B. umbilical artery
C. vitelline vein
D. 3rd aortic arch
E. 6th aortic arch

A. is correct.
The ligamentum teres hepatis is the remnant of the umbilical vein after the umbilical vein closes at birth. It can be found in the falciform ligament, a ventral mesentery derivative.

11.026 Of the following, the one most closely associated with the portal vein is:

A. umbilical vein
B. umbilical artery
C. vitelline vein
D. 3rd aortic arch
E. 6th aortic arch

C. is correct.
The portal vein forms when an anastomotic network around the duodenum forms one vessel. This anastomotic network is from the veins of the gut, the vitelline veins.

11.027 Of the following, the one most closely associated with the common carotid artery is:

A. umbilical vein
B. umbilical artery
C. vitelline vein
D. 3rd aortic arch
E. 6th aortic arch

D. is correct.
The common carotid artery is from the 3rd aortic arch. The 3rd arch also contributes to the proximal internal carotid artery. The external carotid is a branch of the 3rd arch.

11.028 Of the following, the one most closely associated with the ligamentum arteriosum is:

A. umbilical vein
B. umbilical artery
C. vitelline vein
D. 3rd aortic arch
E. 6th aortic arch

E. is correct.
At birth, or shortly thereafter, the ductus arteriosus closes, forming the ligamentum arteriosum. The ductus arteriosus is the distal portion of the left 6th aortic arch and connects the left pulmonary artery with the aorta, to shunt blood away from the nonfunctioning fetal lungs.

11.029 Of the following, the one most closely associated with the medial umbilical ligament is:

A. umbilical vein
B. umbilical artery
C. vitelline vein
D. 3rd aortic arch
E. 6th aortic arch

B. is correct.
When the distal portions of the umbilical arteries close, they become the medial umbilical ligaments on the inner aspect of the anterior abdominal wall. The proximal part of the umbilical artery, from internal iliac, gives off superior vesical branches to the bladder in the adult before becoming ligamentous.

11.030 The truncus ridges may fail to spiral resulting in transposition of the great vessels.

A. true
B. false

A. is correct.
The truncal ridges or swellings are the progenitors of the aorticopulmonary septum within the truncus arteriosus. During development, they spiral, getting the aorta and pulmonary trunks in proper orientation. If they fail to spiral, transposition of the great vessels can occur.

11.031 In the normal fetal circulation, blood from the placenta bypasses the sinusoidal plexus of the liver by way of the ductus venosus.

A. true
B. false

A. is correct.
The ductus venosus is a shunt that develops between the left umbilical vein and the posthepatic inferior vena cava that allows oxygenated blood from the placenta to bypass the liver sinusoids.

11.032 Abnormal origin of the right subclavian artery results from abnormal obliteration of the right 7th intersegmental artery.

A. true
B. false

B. is correct.
The right subclavian artery is normally formed by the right fourth aortic arch, the proximal part of the right dorsal aorta and right 7th intersegmental artery. Abnormal origin of the right subclavian occurs when the proximal right dorsal aorta is obliterated and the distal part persists, creating a retroesophageal right subclavian.

11.033 In aortic valvular atresia, blood passes into the aorta through a patent ductus arteriosus.

A. true
B. false

A. is correct.
In order for a patient with an atretic aortic valve to survive, there must be a patent ductus in order for blood to reach the systemic circulation.

11.034 The valve of the foramen ovale is formed by septum secundum.

A. true
B. false

B. is correct.
The valve of the foramen ovale is formed by the septum primum. As long as the pressure in the pulmonary circuit remains lower than systemic, this valve remains pushed open. However, after birth, the lungs expand, ductus arteriosus closes, pressure in the left atrium increases, and the valve of foramen ovale is pushed closed.

11.035 The least serious clinical problems can be expected from which of the following cardiac abnormalities?

A. patent ductus arteriosus
B. mitral valve stenosis
C. atrial septal defect
D. dextrocardia or right-sided heart

D. is correct.
In the case of dextrocardia, there is transposition so that the heart and great vessels are mirror images of normal. This is a benign situation that is often accompanied by transposition of abdominal viscera, as well. As long as there are no other defects, the patient may never notice the abnormality.

11.036 In tricuspid atresia, there is usually:

A. a patent foramen ovale
B. a ventricular septal defect
C. an underdeveloped right ventricle
D. hypertrophy of the left ventricle
E. all of the above are correct

E. is correct.
With tricuspid atresia, you always see a patent foramen ovale, a ventricular septal defect and underdeveloped right ventricle and a hypertrophic left ventricle.

11.037 Which of the following does NOT characterize atresia of the valve of the pulmonary artery:

A. a patent foramen ovale is the only outlet for blood from the right side of the heart
B. the right ventricle is markedly underdeveloped
C. a patent ductus arteriosus offers a route of blood flow to the lungs
D. there is an overriding aorta

D. is correct.
When the pulmonary valve is atretic, the only way for blood to get out of the right side is via a patent foramen ovale. Conversely, the only way for blood to get to the lungs is via the patent ductus arteriosus. Because the right ventricle is not pumping blood, it becomes markedly hypoplastic. There is no overriding aorta.

11.038 The sinus venosus:

A. has a right horn which persists in the adult as the coronary sinus
B. has a left venous valve which develops into the valve of the coronary sinus
C. forms the smooth-walled portion of the adult right atrium
D. receives blood directly from the portal vein

C. is correct.
The left sinus horn regresses and persists as the main vein of the heart, the coronary sinus, whose valve arises from the inferior part of the right venous valve. The right sinus horn is incorporated into the right atrium, where it forms the smooth-walled part. The portal vein does not send blood to the sinus venosus.

11.039 In the development of the cardiovascular system:

A. angiogenic clusters appear in the yolk sac endoderm
B. the midline heart tube forms four chambers
C. the aortic arches develop in a caudal to cephalic sequence
D. the heart begins to beat around the 21st day

D. is correct.
Angiogenic cell clusters appear in mesoderm only. The heart arises as two bilateral tubes that eventually fuse into one heart tube that begins to beat around the 21st day. When the aortic arches develop, they do so in a cephalic to caudal direction.

11.041 Concerning the truncus ridges, which statement is NOT correct:

A. They may grow abnormally and contribute to formation of transposition of the great vessels
B. They normally spiral around each other as they grow
C. They form the aorticopulmonary septum
D. They contribute to the interatrial septum

D. is correct.
The truncal ridges or swellings are the progenitors of the aorticopulmonary septum within the truncus arteriosus. During development, they spiral, properly orienting the aorta and pulmonary trunks. If they fail to spiral, transposition of the great vessels can occur. They do not involve the interatrial septum.

11.042 Ostium secundum defect:

A. is characterized by a large opening between left and right atria
B. may be caused by excessive resorption of septum primum
C. may be caused by inadequate development of septum secundum
D. may be accompanied by intracardiac shunting of blood
E. all of the above are correct

E. is correct.
An ostium secundum defect is a large opening between the atria that can be caused either by excessive resorption of the septum primum or inadequate development of the septum secundum. Depending on the size of the defect, there can be shunting of the blood between the atria.

11.043 In the development of the heart:

A. the coronary sinus is formed from the left horn of the sinus venosus
B. the oblique vein of the left atrium is formed from the left posterior cardinal vein
C. the valve of the coronary sinus is formed from the left sinus valve
D. the valve of the inferior vena cava is formed from the left sinus valve

A. is correct.
Left horn of sinus venosus forms coronary sinus and left common cardinal vein becomes oblique vein of the left atrium. The right sinus valve becomes the valve of the coronary sinus and the valve of inferior vena cava. Left sinus valve becomes part of interatrial septum.

11.044 The Tetralogy of Fallot includes all of the following EXCEPT:

A. pulmonary stenosis
B. overriding aorta
C. right ventricular hypertrophy
D. atrial septal defect

D. is correct.
The defects in the Tetralogy of Fallot are pulmonary stenosis, ventricular septal defect, overriding aorta and right ventricular hypertrophy. The abnormalities result from abnormal conotruncal septation.

11.045 With aortic valvular atresia:

A. the left atrium and left ventricle are hyperplastic, or overdeveloped
B. there is an overriding aorta
C. blood passes into the aorta through a patent ductus arteriosus
D. blood fails to reach the descending aorta

C. is correct.
In order for a patient with an atretic aortic semilunar valve to survive, there must be a patent ductus arteriosus so that blood can reach the systemic circulation. Because the left ventricle is unable to pump, it is HYPOplastic. There is no overriding aorta.

11.046 Which of the following associations are correct?

A. ligamentum teres hepatis - umbilical vein
B. ligamentum venosum - posterior cardinal v.
C. median umbilical ligaments - umbilical a.
D. ligamentum arteriosum - aortic sac

A. is correct.
The ligamentum teres hepatis is the remnant of the umbilical vein, and it lies within the falciform ligament, formed from the ventral mesentery. The distal parts of the umbilical arteries close and become medial umbilical ligaments. Ductus venosus becomes ligamentum venosum, and ductus arteriosus becomes ligamentum arteriosum.

11.047 In normal fetal circulation:

A. the umbilical arteries carry oxygenated blood from the placenta to the embryo
B. the foramen ovale shunts oxygenated blood from the left to the right side of the heart
C. blood can enter the pulmonary circulation via the ductus arteriosus
D. blood from the placenta bypasses the sinusoidal plexus of the liver in the ductus venosus

D. is correct.
Oxygenated blood from the placenta is carried via the umbilical veins. This blood bypasses the liver sinusoids via the ductus venosus. Upon reaching the heart, oxygenated blood can be shunted from right to left via the foramen ovale. The ductus arteriosus also passes blood from pulmonary to systemic circuits.

11.048 At birth, increased pressure in the left atrium is directly caused by:

A. closure of the foramen ovale
B. cessation of placental blood flow
C. closure of the ductus venosus
D. closure of the ductus arteriosus

D. is correct.
The increased left atrial pressure is directly caused by the closure of the ductus arteriosus, forcing the blood to pass into the lungs and then return in pulmonary veins to the left atrium. The cessation of placental blood flow causes a decrease in systemic pressure and pressure in right atrium, closing foramen ovale.

11.049 Which of the following associations are correct?

A. patent ductus arteriosus - left 6th aortic arch
B. double aortic arch - right dorsal aorta
C. common carotid artery - 3rd aortic arch
D. double superior vena cava - left anterior cardinal vein
E. all of the above are correct

E. is correct.
A patent ductus involves the left 6th arch. A double aortic arch is caused by persistence of the right dorsal aorta. The common carotid artery is a derivative of the 3rd arch. A double superior vena cava is caused by persistence of part of the left anterior cardinal vein.

11.050 Partitioning of the atrium is accomplished by growth of:

A. septum primum
B. septum secundum
C. both
D. neither

C. is correct.
The growth of both the septum primum and septum secundum contribute to the partitioning of the atrium. Septum primum grows down to meet the endocardial heart cushions, closing foramen primum. Foramen secundum forms within septum primum, and it will be overlapped by the downgrowth of septum secundum, leaving open foramen ovale.

11.051 Features of the Tetralogy of Fallot include:

A. interatrial septal defect
B. stenosis of the pulmonary artery
C. both
D. neither

B. is correct.
The defects in the Tetralogy of Fallot are pulmonary stenosis, ventricular septal defect, overriding aorta and right ventricular hypertrophy. The tetralogy results from unequal division of the truncus arteriosus and conus cordis. Neural crest is important in this septation event.

11.052 At birth, the distal branches of both internal iliac arteries collapse and persist as the:

A. urachus
B. lateral umbilical ligaments
C. both
D. neither

D. is correct.
When the distal parts of the umbilical arteries collapse at birth, they form the medial umbilical ligaments. The urachus persists as the median umbilical ligament. The lateral umbilical folds are peritoneum overlying the inferior epigastric vessels.

11.053 The mesenchymal cells which aggregate to form blood islands are called:

A. hemoblasts
B. mesoblasts
C. fibroblasts
D. angioblasts
E. none of the above

D. is correct.
Angioblasts are the cells that form the blood islands. These blood islands then develop into the blood cells and the endothelium of the blood vessels. This early blood cell and blood vessel formation occurs first in the extraembryonic mesoderm of the yolk sac, chorion and connecting stalk.

11.054 Closure of the foramen primum results from fusion of the:

A. septum secundum and the fused endocardial cushions
B. septum secundum and the septum primum
C. septum primum and the fused endocardial cushions
D. septum primum and the septum spurium
E. septum primum and the sinoatrial valves

C. is correct.
The septum primum and the endocardial cushions fuse to close the foramen primum. Subsequently, perforations in the upper part of the septum primum coalesce to form the foramen secundum. It is this foramen that closes postnatally when left atrial pressure equals right atrial pressure.

11.055 The most common type of cardiac septal defect is:

A. muscular type ventricular septal defect, or VSD
B. secundum type atrial septal defect, or ASD
C. membranous type VSD
D. primum type ASD
E. sinus venosus

C. is correct.
Although the most common ATRIAL septal defect is the secundum type ASD, the overall most common cardiac septal defect is the membranous type VSD.

11.056 Congenital heart disease is the most common cardiac condition in childhood and most frequently results from:

A. maternal medication
B. mutant genes
C. rubella virus
D. fetal distress
E. genetic and environmental factors

E. is correct.
The causes of congenital heart disease are vast and varied. The term "genetic and environmental factors" is a good blanket term that covers all the possibilities. Rubella, an environmental influence, is known to cause heart defects. Heart defects are found in a number of heritable syndromes.

11.057 The fetal left atrium is mainly derived from the:

A. primitive pulmonary vein
B. primitive atrium
C. right pulmonary vein
D. sinus venarum
E. sinus venosus

A. is correct.
The primitive pulmonary vein becomes incorporated into the wall of the fetal left atrium, forming most of it. The original left atrium becomes a trabeculated atrial appendage called the left auricle, because it resembles an "ear" on the heart.

11.058 The fetal right atrium is mainly derived from:

A. primitive pulmonary vein
B. primitive atrium
C. right pulmonary vein
D. sinus venarum
E. sinus venosus

E. is correct.
The right sinus horn of the sinus venosus enlarges and forms the fetal right atrium. The left sinus horn regresses to form the main vein draining the heart muscle, the coronary sinus. The original right atrium becomes the right auricle and also part of right atrium anterior to the crista terminalis.

11.059 The most common congenital malformation of the great vessels is:

A. coarctation of the aorta
B. Tetralogy of Fallot
C. patent ductus arteriosus
D. persistent left superior vena cava
E. pulmonary semilunar valve stenosis

C. is correct.
Patent ductus arteriosus is the most common congenital malformation of the great vessels. The ductus arteriosus is the distal portion of the left sixth aortic arch that connects the left pulmonary artery to the aorta.

11.060 Neural crest forms the walls of the great vessels, but not the endothelium of those vessels.

A. true
B. false

A. is correct.
Neural crest is very important in heart development. In addition to providing the mechanism behind conotruncal septation, neural crest populates the walls of the great vessels and forms smooth muscle there.

11.061 The oblique vein of the left atrium is a remnant of the left common cardinal vein.

A. true
B. false

A. is correct.
Common cardinal veins drain anterior & posterior cardinal veins to sinus venosus. Left sinus horn becomes coronary vein. Left common cardinal becomes oblique vein of the left atrium. A remnant of left anterior cardinal, ligament of the left superior vena cava, connects oblique vein to left superior intercostal & brachiocephalic veins.

11.062 The bulbar portion of the developing heart is incorporated such as to form most of the left ventricle.

A. true
B. false

B. is correct.
The bulbus cordis of the primitive heart tube leads from the single primitive ventricle into conus cordis and truncus arteriosus. The bending of the heart creates the bulboventricular sulcus, which separates bulbus, destined to become right ventricle, from primitive ventricle, destined to become left ventricle.

11.063 The conus of the heart forms infundibulum of the right ventricle and aortic vestibule of the left ventricle.

A. true
B. false

A. is correct.
Conus cordis connects bulbus cordis, future right ventricle, with truncus arteriosus. Truncus is divided by a spiralling septum into ascending aorta and pulmonary trunk, while conus is divided into the outflow regions of both ventricles, infundibulum & aortic vestibule.

11.064 To adequately form the outflow of the heart, the aortic sac, the truncus arteriosus and the conus cordis must all be septated, and neural crest cells play a major role in this septation.

A. true
B. false

A. is correct.
The outflow region of the heart is septated by migration of neural crest cells. Aortic sac, from which aortic arches branch, becomes proximal adult aortic arch & brachiocephalic trunk. Truncus becomes ascending aorta & pulmonary trunk, while conus becomes infundibulum and aortic vestibule.

11.065 The remnant of the first aortic arch artery is:
- A. stapedial artery
- B. internal carotid artery
- C. maxillary artery
- D. common carotid artery
- E. the 1st arch artery regresses without remnants

C. is correct.
First arch becomes maxillary; 2nd arch remnants are stapedial and hyoid arteries; 3rd arch becomes common & proximal internal carotid arteries; 4th arch becomes proximal right subclavian & part of arch of aorta; 6th arch becomes proximal pulmonary arteries and ductus arteriosus.

11.066 The left brachiocephalic vein is derived from:
- A. left anterior cardinal vein
- B. left posterior cardinal vein
- C. a shunt between left and right posterior cardinal veins
- D. left horn of the sinus venosus
- E. none of the above

E. is correct.
The cranial end of left brachiocephalic vein is from left anterior cardinal, but the lower part develops as a shunt between left and right anterior cardinal veins. On the right side, the upper part of superior vena cava is from right anterior cardinal, while the lower part is old right common cardinal vein.

11.067 The aortic sac:
- A. is the area immediately distal to the ventricles
- B. is connected to the dorsal aorta via the aortic arch arteries
- C. is preserved as the region of the semilunar valves in the adult heart
- D. is also known as the truncus arteriosus
- E. none of the above

B. is correct.
The aortic sac receives blood from the truncus arteriosus and sends it into the aortic arch arteries which branch from it and connect it to the paired dorsal aortae. Aortic sac becomes the proximal part of aortic arch & the brachiocephalic trunk. Semilunar valves arise from the walls of truncus arteriosus.

11.068 The crista terminalis is derived from:
- A. right horn of the sinus venosus
- B. left horn of the sinus venosus
- C. primitive atrium
- D. AV canal
- E. right cusp of the valve of the sinus venosus

E. is correct.
This is pretty picky. Crista terminalis is the ridge on the inner surface of the right atrium that demarcates the smooth walled part derived from sinus venosus and the pectinate muscle-containing part from primitive right atrium. It marks where the right cusp of the sinoatrial valve was before the sinus became part of atrium.

11.069 The membranous portion of the interventricular septum is formed by:
- A. conal ridges
- B. truncal ridges
- C. endocardial cushions
- D. septum primum
- E. more than one of the above

E. is correct.
The posterosuperior portion of the interventricular septum is the membranous portion. It is formed by the fusion of the conal or bulbar ridges with the endocardial cushions and the muscular portion of interventricular septum. Truncal ridges are up in truncus, and septum primum helps to divide the atria.

11.070 The region of the atrioventricular canal develops into:
- A. the semilunar valves
- B. the atrial septum
- C. the mitral and tricuspid valves
- D. the base of the ventricle
- E. the trabeculated portion of the right atrium

C. is correct.
With a name like atrioventricular canal, you might hope it would become something to do with the atrioventricular valves. The single canal is divided by the ingrowth of the endocardial cushions. The right atrioventricular valve is the tricuspid, while the left AV valve is bicuspid, known as the mitral valve.

11.071 The myocardial layer of the heart tube develops from:

A. the endocardial tubes
B. dorsal mesocardium
C. cardiac jelly
D. splanchnic mesoderm
E. septum transversum

D. is correct.
Myocardium or heart muscle arises from the splanchnic mesoderm near the heart tubes in the cardiogenic region. Endocardium is also from this cardiogenic splanchnic mesoderm, from angiogenic cell clusters forming the heart tubes. Epicardium or visceral pericardium is from splanchnic mesoderm lining the intraembryonic coelom.

11.072 The cardiac jelly:

A. separates the endocardium from the myocardium
B. mediates interactions between endocardium and myocardium
C. resembles a thick basement membrane
D. becomes the subendocardial connective tissue layer of the heart
E. all of the above

E. is correct.
Cardiac jelly is a relatively thick layer of extracellular matrix material that lies between endocardium and myocardium during early heart formation. As with extracellular matrix in many places, it is suspected of involvement in cellular interactions during heart development.

11.073 The epicardium forms from:

A. the epimyocardial layer of the heart
B. dorsal mesocardium over the sinus venosus
C. cardiogenic plate mesoderm
D. the endocardium
E. none of the above

A. is correct.
The epimyocardial layer of the developing heart develops from the splanchnic mesoderm between heart tubes and the intraembryonic coelom in the cardiogenic area. The part of the epimyocardium that lines this region of the coelom becomes visceral serous pericardium while mesoderm between this and the heart tubes becomes myocardium.

11.074 The arch of the azygos vein is derived from:

A. posterior cardinal vein
B. anterior cardinal vein
C. common cardinal vein
D. supracardinal vein
E. subcardinal vein

A. is correct.
The azygos system of veins are indirect descendants of the posterior cardinal veins, although arch of the azygos is old right posterior cardinal. The point at which azygos arch empties into superior vena cava in the adult marks the junction of old anterior cardinal above with old common cardinal below.

11.075 Which structure is most important in the formation of the valve of the foramen ovale?

A. ductus arteriosus
B. ductus venosus
C. endocardial cushion
D. septum primum
E. septum secundum
F. dorsal mesocardium
G. truncus arteriosus
H. truncal ridges
I. bulbus cordis
J. sinus venosus
K. bulboventricular ridge
L. cardiac jelly

E. is correct.
The ostium secundum is nearly closed by the growth of the septum secundum, which forms the valve of the foramen ovale. This remains patent until birth, allowing blood to be shunted from right to left atrium. After birth, the closing of ductus arteriosus forces blood into the pulmonary circuit, and the returning blood fills left atrium, balancing the pressure in the right atrium and closing the valve of the foramen ovale.

11.076 Which of the following structures ruptures to create the transverse pericardial sinus?

A. ductus arteriosus
B. ductus venosus
C. endocardial cushion
D. septum primum
E. septum secundum
F. dorsal mesocardium
G. truncus arteriosus
H. truncal ridges
I. bulbus cordis
J. sinus venosus
K. bulboventricular ridge
L. cardiac jelly

F. is correct.
Early in heart development, the heart tubes are suspended within the intraembryonic coelom by the dorsal mesocardium. The rupture of this membrane and the folding of the heart tubes brings the outflow tract and inflow tract close together, producing the transverse pericardial sinus.

11.077 Transposition of the great vessels is most directly related to abnormal development of which of the following?

A. ductus arteriosus
B. ductus venosus
C. endocardial cushion
D. septum primum
E. septum secundum
F. dorsal mesocardium
G. truncus arteriosus
H. truncal ridge
I. bulbus cordis
J. sinus venosus
K. bulboventricular ridge
L. cardiac jelly

H. is correct.
The spiral aorticopulmonary septum forms within the truncus arteriosus as the result of the growth of the truncal swellings or ridges.

11.078 Which structure is important for atrial and ventricular septum formation, as well as formation of the artioventricular valves?

A. ductus arteriosus
B. ductus venosus
C. endocardial cushion
D. septum primum
E. septum secundum
F. dorsal mesocardium
G. truncus arteriosus
H. truncal ridges
I. bulbus cordis
J. sinus venosus
K. bulboventricular ridge
L. cardiac jelly

C. is correct.
The endocardial cushions are centrally located within the developing heart, and they are involved in the development of several heart structures, including the interatrial septum, membranous portion of the interventricular septum, the artioventricular valves, and the aorticopulmonary septum.

SECTION 12: RESPIRATORY AND DIGESTIVE SYSTEM

12.001 The stage of lung development, 6 mos. to after birth, during which the respiratory epithelium becomes squamous and the capillary loops are intimately related to the epithelium is the:

A. glandular period
B. vascular period
C. alveolar period
D. canalicular period
E. acinar period

C. is correct.
Lung development may be divided into four overlapping stages: pseudoglandular period, from 5-17wks; canalicular period, from 16-25 wks; terminal sac period, 24 wks-birth; alveolar period, 6 mos-8 yrs. It is during this last period that the epithelium flattens and alveoli proliferate, allowing gas exchange.

12.002 In the development of the lung, which of the following is NOT correct:

A. alveolar collapse in hyaline membrane disease is a result of insufficient surfactant production
B. alveoli continue to form postnatally
C. alveoli contain specialized epithelial cells which produce surfactant
D. alveolar epithelium is derived from splanchnic mesoderm

D. is correct.
Alveoli continue to form after birth, with only 1/8 to 1/6 of the adult alveoli present in the newborn. Alveoli have type II pneumocyte cells producing surfactant. Premature infants often make insufficient surfactant, causing hyaline membrane disease. Epithelium of the lungs is from the endoderm.

12.003 Meckel's diverticulum is an adult remnant of the:

A. urachus
B. hindgut
C. pars cystica
D. vitelline duct
E. dorsal pancreatic duct

D. is correct.
Vitelline duct is a connection between embryonic midgut and yolk sac, from which gut developed. As development proceeds, vitelline duct normally regresses. If it does not, it may persist as a Meckel's diverticulum, a vitelline duct cyst, an umbilical/vitelline fistula, or a fibrous cord connecting gut to umbilicus.

12.004 Endodermal derivatives of the gut include:

A. gallbladder muscle
B. liver hepatocytes
C. ligament of Treitz
D. gastric luminal epithelium
E. more than one of the above

E. is correct.
The liver hepatocytes and gastric luminal epithelium are endodermal derivatives of the gut. The gallbladder muscle, like all muscle, is mesodermal. The ligament of Treitz or suspensory ligament of the duodenum is also mesodermal, because it is derived from the right crus of the diaphragm, a mesodermal structure.

12.005 The endodermal hepatic diverticulum does NOT give rise to:

A. part of the pancreas
B. gallbladder
C. epithelial part of the liver
D. ductus venosus

D. is correct.
The endoderm that buds out as the hepatic diverticulum ultimately differentiates into the parenchyma of the liver, the gallbladder and the ventral pancreatic bud. The ductus venosus is mesodermal, because it is a blood vessel.

12.006 The following events in the development of the abdominal cavity are greatly affected by the rapid growth of the liver:

A. urorectal septum formation
B. dorsal mesentery morphogenesis
C. formation of inferior recess of lesser sac
D. herniation of midgut loop

D. is correct.
The rapid growth of the liver has considerable effect on the development of the ventral mesentery, and it promotes the herniation of the midgut by occupying space in the abdominal cavity. It does not affect urorectal septum formation or the inferior recess of the lesser sac.

12.007 Factors, major events, or structures associated with midgut development include:

A. 270 degree rotation
B. rapid growth of cranial limb
C. vitelline duct
D. 3rd part of the duodenum
E. all of the above are correct

E. is correct.
The midgut begins immediately distal to where the bile duct enters the duodenum. During development, it is characterized by 270 degree rotation, by herniation into the umbilicus in which the cranial limb grows most rapidly, and by attachment of the vitelline duct to the apex of the herniating loop.

12.008 In its development, the stomach does NOT:

A. rotate 90 degrees clockwise when viewed from above
B. descend
C. exhibit differential growth
D. cause ventral mesentery development

D. is correct.
During its development, the stomach makes a 90 degree rotation clockwise. Different areas of the stomach also grow at different rates, giving it its characteristic shape. Stomach descends as the esophagus grows in length, explaining why thoracic splanchnic nerves to the gut arise from sympathetic ganglia T5-12.

12.009 The embryonic foregut differentiates into all or part of the:

A. liver
B. ventral pancreas
C. esophagus
D. lung
E. all of the above are correct

E. is correct.
Derivatives of embryonic foregut include pharynx, esophagus, lungs & respiratory tract, stomach, the part of the duodenum cranial to the hepatic diverticulum, the pancreas, liver and gall bladder.

12.010 The allantois is derived from:

A. ectoderm
B. endoderm
C. both
D. neither

B. is correct.
The allantois is an endodermal outpouching of the yolk sac. Early on, it is attached to the hindgut, but when the urorectal septum divides the cloaca, it becomes associated with the urinary bladder and contributes to its development. The allantois forms the urachus and then the median umbilical ligament.

12.011 The cloacal membrane is derived from:

A. ectoderm
B. endoderm
C. both
D. neither

C. is correct.
The cloacal membrane and prochordal plate are the two places in the embryo where ectoderm and endoderm remain in apposition, after the formation of mesoderm from the primitive streak. Therefore, the cloacal membrane consists of both layers.

12.012 The vermiform appendix arises from:

A. endoderm
B. mesoderm
C. both
D. neither

C. is correct.
The vermiform appendix is an outgrowth of the midgut in the region of the cecum. Like the rest of the gut, it is an endodermally-lined cavity that has a muscular wall derived from mesoderm.

12.013 The liver is a derivative of:
A. the embryonic foregut
B. the embryonic midgut
C. both
D. neither

A. is correct.
The embryonic foregut gives rise to pharynx, esophagus, lungs and respiratory tract, stomach, the part of the duodenum cranial to the hepatic bud, pancreas, liver and gall bladder.

12.014 The spleen is a derivative of:
A. the embryonic foregut
B. the embryonic midgut
C. both
D. neither

D. is correct.
The spleen, although it develops in the dorsal mesogastrium, is not a derivative of the gut. It is hemopoietic tissue that is actually more a part of the circulatory system. It develops from mesenchyme within the dorsal mesogastrium. Spleen also has a role in the development of the immune system in the fetus & neonate.

12.015 The vermiform appendix is a derivative of:
A. the embryonic foregut
B. the embryonic midgut
C. both
D. neither

B. is correct.
The vermiform appendix is an outgrowth of the midgut in the region of the cecum. Like the rest of the gut, it is an endodermally lined cavity that has a muscular wall derived from mesoderm. Following the rotation of the gut, appendix comes to lie, usually, in the iliac fossa.

12.016 Abnormal intestinal rotation during fetal development may produce the following:
A. congenital umbilical hernia
B. annular pancreas
C. infarction and gangrene
D. diaphragmatic hernia
E. Meckel's diverticulum or diverticulum ilei

C. is correct.
Abnormal rotation of the intestinal loop causes it to return to the abdomen in a different order, with the colon being the first to return to the gut. This positions things backwards, and the gut may twist abnormally. Such twisting or volvulus can obstruct the blood supply to the gut, resulting in infarction and gangrene.

12.017 An umbilical fistula is associated with:
A. allantoic duct
B. vitelline duct
C. both
D. neither

C. is correct.
A fistula involving the umbilicus may involve either the allantoic or vitelline duct. A vitelline fistula is a patent vitelline duct connecting the umbilicus to the midgut, so there may be fecal discharge at the umbilicus. A urachal fistula connects to the bladder, so there may be some urine at the umbilicus.

12.018 The round ligament of the liver, or ligamentum teres hepatis, is associated with:
A. allantoic duct
B. vitelline duct
C. both
D. neither

D. is correct.
The ligamentum teres hepatis is the remnant of the umbilical vein. Don't confuse this with ligamentum teres uteri, or round ligament of the uterus, which is a remnant of the gubernaculum.

12.019 Meckel's diverticulum is associated with:
A. allantoic duct
B. vitelline duct
C. both
D. neither

B. is correct.
Meckel's diverticulum is the persistence of the vitelline duct as an outpouching of the ileum. It is usually unnoticed, but may become inflamed. It may also contain ectopic pancreatic or gastric tissue that can cause ulceration, hemorrhage and perforation.

12.020 All of us has "suffered" which one of the following types of hernia?

A. inguinal
B. umbilical
C. lumbar
D. diaphragmatic
E. femoral

B. is correct.
The herniation of the midgut out through the umbilicus is a normal event in development. However, the intestinal contents may fail to return to the abdomen, resulting in an omphalocoele. Viscera may herniate later through the weak umbilical region, and this is a true umbilical hernia.

12.021 During the development of the gut:

A. the pancreas receives part of its blood supply via the celiac trunk
B. the stomach rotates, causing the left vagal trunk to innervate its posterior wall
C. the urorectal fold may fail to divide the cloaca, causing a rectouterine fistula in the female
D. the transverse colon becomes retroperitoneal

A. is correct.
Pancreas is a derivative of the caudal foregut, so it receives blood from the celiac trunk. The rotation of the stomach is such that the left vagal trunk innervates its anterior wall. A urorectal fistula results from failure of the urorectal fold to divide the cloaca. The transverse colon remains intraperitoneal.

12.022 In the digestive system:

A. endoderm forms the lining of the stomach and lung and the parenchymal cells of the liver
B. gut rotation and fusion of mesentery to the dorsal body wall makes the spleen retroperitoneal
C. the duodenum is supplied by both superior and inferior mesenteric artery
D. the inferior mesenteric artery is the axis for counterclockwise rotation of the midgut loop

A. is correct.
Endoderm lines the gut and lungs and forms the liver parenchyma. The spleen remains intraperitoneal. The duodenum, being of both foregut and midgut origin, receives blood from both the celiac trunk and the superior mesenteric artery. The superior mesenteric artery is the axis of rotation of the midgut.

12.023 In the digestive system:

A. failure of the intestinal loops to return into the abdominal cavity forms Meckel's diverticulum
B. an omphalocele would most likely develop around the 10th-12th week of gestation
C. stenosis of the gut most frequently occurs in the large intestine
D. an annular pancreas is caused by a failure in normal migration of the dorsal pancreas

B. is correct.
Return of the intestinal loops to the abdomen occurs toward the end of the third month. Failure to do so results in an omphalocoele. Stenosis of the gut is most common in the duodenum. An annular pancreas results when the left portion of the ventral pancreas migrates in a direction opposite normal.

12.024 The developing liver does NOT:

A. contain cells derived from mesoderm
B. have a hemopoietic function in the fetus
C. have a gall bladder derived from the hepatic diverticulum
D. have hepatic sinusoids which receive the majority of their blood from the left umbilical vein

D. is correct.
The parenchyma of the liver is endodermal, but there are mesodermal hemopoietic, phagocytic and connective tissue cells. The gall bladder is from the hepatic diverticulum. The main blood supply to the sinusoids is the portal vein. The blood from the left umbilical vein bypasses the sinusoids via the ductus venosus.

12.025 Which of the following conditions would most likely cause vomiting in the newborn?

A. umbilical fistula
B. duodenal stenosis
C. rectal atresia
D. stenosis of the transverse colon

B. is correct.
Vomiting would most likely be caused by an obstruction in the upper part of the GI tract. Esophageal atresia or duodenal stenosis could cause this.

12.026 During development of the gut:

A. the stomach rotates, so that the greater curvature faces to the left and inferiorly
B. retention of the vitelline duct may produce an umbilical fistula
C. the urorectal septum may fail to divide the cloaca, causing a rectovaginal fistula in the female
D. the descending colon becomes retroperitoneal
E. all of the above are correct

E. is correct.
Following rotation of the stomach, the lesser curvature faces to the right and superiorly, while the greater curvature faces left and inferiorly. Persistence of the vitelline duct may cause umbilical fistula. Rupture of the urorectal septum can produce rectovaginal fistula. Ascending & descending colon are retroperitoneal.

12.027 In the development of the gut:

A. the celiac trunk represents the blood supply to the midgut
B. the early embryo maintains a connection between the midgut and the yolk sac via the allantois
C. muscle, connective tissue and blood vessels in the gut wall are derived from splanchnic mesoderm
D. the primitive gut tube is in open communication with the amniotic cavity

C. is correct.
The foregut is supplied by the celiac trunk. The embryonic midgut connects with the yolk sac via the vitelline duct. Splanchnic mesoderm contributes to the mesodermal components of the gut wall. The gut communicates with amniotic cavity after the 4th week, when the oropharyngeal membrane ruptures.

12.028 Gut rotations and subsequent fusion of mesentery to the dorsal body wall causes which of the following to assume a retroperitoneal position?

A. gall bladder
B. pancreas
C. spleen
D. jejunum

B. is correct.
Due to gut rotation and mesentery fusions, most of the pancreas and duodenum and the ascending and descending colons become secondarily retroperitoneal.

12.029 In the formation of the pancreas:

A. a dorsal and ventral bud from the endoderm of the duodenum are the first indications of a pancreas
B. the ventral pancreatic bud degenerates
C. an annular pancreas forms if a portion of the dorsal bud rotates abnormally
D. insulin is not secreted during fetal life

A. is correct.
Pancreas forms from endodermal diverticula from the hepatic bud and the duodenum. The ventral bud develops into the uncinate process, but if it rotates abnormally it can cause an annular pancreas. Insulin secretion begins around the 5th month of development.

12.030 The liver:
- A. receives blood from the placenta via the umbilical vein which runs in the falciform ligament
- B. forms as a diverticulum from the foregut endoderm
- C. contains hemopoietic and connective tissue cells derived from mesoderm of the septum transversum
- D. contains hepatic sinusoids derived from the vitelline veins
- E. all of the above are correct

E. is correct.
Liver develops from an endodermal hepatic diverticulum, but also contains mesodermal hemopoietic & connective tissue. Blood from the placenta reaches liver via the left umbilical vein but by-passes the sinusoids through the ductus venosus. The sinusoids are derived from the vitelline veins.

12.031 In the development of the midgut:
- A. the superior mesenteric artery is the axis for clockwise rotation of the midgut loop
- B. the persistence of part of the vitelline duct leads to urachal fistula
- C. a vitelline cyst may result from abnormal remodelling of the vitelline veins
- D. an omphalocele is not synonymous with congenital umbilical hernia

D. is correct.
The midgut rotates in a counterclockwise direction around superior mesenteric artery. Persistence of the vitelline duct may cause a vitelline fistula or cyst. Omphalocele results from a failure of midgut to return to the abdominal cavity, while congenital umbilical hernia is a later herniation of gut through abdominal wall.

12.032 The yolk sac detaches from the gut by the end of the:
- A. 2nd week
- B. 5th week
- C. 3rd month
- D. 4th month
- E. 5th month

B. is correct.
Through body folding, the yolk sac separates from the gut during the 5th week, although the gut remains attached to the yolk sac by the vitelline duct, which persists into the third month of development.

12.033 A persistence of the vitelline duct may result in:
- A. ileal diverticulum
- B. Meckel's diverticulum
- C. vitelline cyst
- D. umbilical fistula
- E. all of the above

E. is correct.
If the vitelline duct remains patent, there will be an umbilical or vitelline fistula, leaking meconium or fetal feces at the umbilicus. Partial closure of vitelline duct may result in a vitelline cyst or a Meckel's/ileal diverticulum. The latter are found on the anti-mesenteric side of ileum within 2 feet of cecum.

12.034 During embryological development, the large intestine is:
- A. last to leave the umbilical cord and re-enter the abdominal cavity
- B. always longer than the small intestine
- C. both
- D. neither

A. is correct.
The large intestine is normally the last to leave the umbilical cord to return to the abdomen. However, abnormal rotation of the midgut can cause it to return first, creating a left-sided colon. Rapid growth of the small intestine makes it much longer than the large intestine.

12.035 Typical bile, secreted by hepatic cells:
- A. occurs in fetuses 5 months old
- B. colors the meconium
- C. both
- D. neither

C. is correct.
Bile production begins around the 12th week of development, so it would occur during the 5th month. The bile gives the meconium a greenish color. Meconium is the fecal material of the fetus.

12.036 Accessory pancreases:

A. are extremely rare
B. occur within the wall of the intestine and stomach
C. both
D. neither

B. is correct.
Heterotopic pancreatic tissue is fairly common. It will usually occur in the mucosa of the stomach or in a Meckel's diverticulum.

12.037 Factors assisting in the rotation of the stomach include:

A. rapid expansion of the dorsal mesentery
B. slow growth of the ventral mesentery
C. both
D. neither

C. is correct.
The rapid expansion of the dorsal mesentery and slow growth of the ventral mesentery both contribute to the rotation of the stomach.

12.038 The terminal dilated part of the hindgut is called the:

A. cloaca
B. yolk stalk
C. allantois
D. cecum
E. coelom

A. is correct.
The folding of the embryo brings the allantois and the hindgut into association. The dilated terminal part of the hindgut is called the cloaca, and it communicates with the allantois. Later in development the cloaca is divided by the urorectal septum into the primitive urogenital sinus and the anorectal canal.

12.039 Which of the following arteries supply derivatives of the caudal portion of the foregut?

A. celiac trunk
B. inferior mesenteric artery
C. pulmonary artery
D. umbilical artery
E. common iliac artery

A. is correct.
Celiac trunk is the artery of the caudal portion of the foregut, supplying the stomach, liver, gall bladder, pancreas and upper portion of the duodenum. The superior mesenteric is considered the artery of the midgut, and inferior mesenteric is considered the artery of the hindgut.

12.040 Which of the following statements about the developing duodenum is NOT true?

A. it is a derivative of the foregut and the midgut
B. the yolk stalk is attached to the apex of the duodenal loop
C. it is supplied by branches of the foregut and midgut arteries
D. it becomes C-shaped as it develops and the stomach rotates
E. its lumen is temporarily obliterated by epithelial cells

B. is correct.
During development, it is the MIDGUT to which the yolk stalk or vitelline duct is attached. Duodenum is both foregut & midgut in origin, so both celiac & superior mesenteric arteries supply it. During duodenal development, epithelial growth temporarily closes its lumen.

12.041 The following embryonic structures can give origin to cysts, diverticula, or fistulae in postnatal life EXCEPT:

A. vitelline duct
B. urachus (allantoic duct)
C. ductus venosus (Botalli)
D. neural tube
E. metanephros

C. is correct.
Meckel's diverticulum is from the vitelline duct. Urachal fistula is a persistent allantoic duct. Cystic kidney results from failure of the collecting ducts to meet the metanephric blastema. Spina bifida cystica is a herniation of the spinal cord through a defective vertebral arch. I'd put my money on ductus venosus.

12.042 One-eighth to one-sixth of the adult number of alveoli are present in the lungs at birth. Their numbers increase after birth at least until _____ years of age.

A. 1
B. 2
C. 4
D. 6
E. 8

E. is correct.
The alveolar period of lung development begins during the late fetal period and continues through eight years of age. Approximately 95% of alveoli develop after birth. The alveolar period is also characterized by thinning of the epithelial alveolar lining and the production of surfactant, important in protecting the epithelium.

12.043 Pulmonary surfactant most likely begins to form in the human fetus at about _____ weeks.

A. 16
B. 20
C. 25
D. 30
E. 34

C. is correct.
Surfactant production begins during the terminal sac period of lung development, which is 24 weeks until birth. Although surfactant production begins at this time, the final few weeks of development see a sharp rise in production, preparing the lungs for birth. Insufficient surfactant causes hyaline membrane disease.

12.044 As the stomach acquires its adult shape, it rotates around its longitudinal axis. Which of the following events does not result from this rotation?

A. the ventral border of the stomach moves to the right
B. the dorsal border moves to the left
C. the dorsal mesogastrium is carried to the left
D. the duodenum rotates to the right
E. the dorsal part of the stomach grows more rapidly

E. is correct.
During stomach rotation, the original ventral border comes to face to the right & superiorly while the original dorsal border comes to face left & inferiorly. Duodenum rotates to the right, and dorsal mesogastrium is carried to the left. It is true that the dorsal border of stomach grows more rapidly, but this is not related.

12.045 The pectinate line of the anus marks the junction of:

A. skin and mucous membrane
B. splanchnic and somatic mesoderm
C. ectoderm derivatives and endodermal derivatives
D. old amniotic cavity and yolk sac
E. all of the above are correct

E. is correct.
The pectinate line marks the position of the anal membrane, one of the descendants of the cloacal membrane. Early in development, cloacal membrane, a fusion of ectoderm and endoderm, separates the amniotic cavity from the yolk sac. Yolk sac forms the gut, and the walls of the gut develop from splanchnic mesoderm.

12.046 The muscular wall of the esophagus arises from:

A. somatic mesoderm
B. neural crest
C. branchial arch VI
D. lining of the yolk sac

C. is correct.
The muscle of the upper portion of the esophagus is skeletal muscle, derived from branchial arch VI and innervated by recurrent laryngeal branches of vagus nerve, X. The lower part of the esophageal wall is smooth muscle from splanchnic mesoderm, like the rest of the gut wall. It is innervated by parasympathetics from vagus.

12.047 Which of the following is NOT associated with esophageal atresia:

A. tracheoesophageal fistula
B. polyhydramnios
C. deviation of the tracheoesophageal septum
D. reflux of milk through nose and mouth, which appears toward the end of the first week after birth

D. is correct.
Esophageal atresia is thought to result in some cases by abnormal formation of the tracheoesophageal septum. This also explains why esophageal atresia and tracheoesophageal fistula are often seen together. Polyhydramnios results from lack of fetal swallowing. Reflux of milk occurs immediately upon first ingestion.

12.048 The terminal sac stage of lung development is characterized by the appearance of:

A. secondary bronchi
B. tertiary bronchi
C. respiratory bronchi
D. surfactant
E. mature alveoli

D. is correct.
Tertiary or segmental bronchi are formed by the 8th week. By the end of the canalicular period, at 24 weeks, respiratory bronchi have begun to form. The following stage of lung development, terminal sac stage, involves proliferation of terminal sacs and initiation of surfactant production. Mature alveoli appear after birth.

12.049 The tracheoesophageal septum separates the:

A. laryngotracheal tube and nasopharynx
B. esophagus and nasopharynx
C. laryngotracheal tube and esophagus
D. laryngotracheal tube and oropharynx
E. esophagus and oropharynx

C. is correct.
Pharynx is the common food/air tube, so it would not be wise to put a septum between pharynx and esophagus or trachea. However, the lungs bud from the foregut as an anterior diverticulum between the 4th & 6th branchial arches, explaining why superior laryngeal and recurrent laryngeal nerves from vagus innervate larynx.

12.050 The connective tissues of the lungs develop from splanchnic mesoderm.

A. true
B. false

A. is correct.
The lung bud grows into and branches within the splanchnic mesoderm anterior to foregut. Lungs are lined with endoderm from the foregut but the smooth muscle, cartilage and connective tissue of the lungs develops from splanchnic mesoderm. As the lungs grow, they push into the pericardioperitoneal canals, forming pleural cavities.

12.051 The laryngotracheal diverticulum develops within the floor of the pharynx between arches:

A. I and II
B. II and III
C. III and IV
D. IV and VI
E. none of the above

D. is correct.
The lung bud or laryngotracheal diverticulum buds ventrally from the foregut between branchial arches IV and VI. The nerve of these arches is the vagus, therefore the laryngeal muscles are innervated by branches of X. External branch of superior laryngeal reaches cricothyroid, while recurrent laryngeal does all others.

12.052 The omental apron of the greater omentum:

A. communicates with the peritoneal cavity via the epiploic foramen of Winslow
B. becomes retroperitoneal in the adult
C. has the ascending colon located within its superior boundary
D. is a quadruple layer of peritoneum
E. is lost during embryonic development

D. is correct.
The omental apron is the portion of the greater omentum, continuous with gastrocolic ligament, which hangs from the transverse colon. Early in development, it is an open sac, communicating with the lesser sac or omental bursa. The walls of the sac are two layers of peritoneum, forming a quadruple layer when the bag fuses.

12.053 Which of the following statements concerning the development of the duodenum is FALSE?

A. the duodenum rotates to the right side of the embryo during development
B. most of the duodenum becomes retroperitoneal during development
C. the duodenum develops only from the caudal foregut
D. there is no lumen within the duodenum at some point in development
E. none of the above is false

C. is correct.
Duodenum develops from caudal foregut and cranial midgut. Except for the short first part and end of the fourth part, the duodenum becomes retroperitoneal after rotating to the right. Epithelial overgrowth temporarily obliterates the duodenal lumen, and duodenal stenosis or atresia may result from failed recanalization.

12.054 Which of the following structures is most closely related to the development of the cloaca?

A. liver
B. stomach
C. spleen
D. duodenum
E. pancreas
F. gall bladder
G. jejunum
H. ileum
I. cecum
J. appendix
K. ascending colon
L. transverse colon
M. descending colon
N. sigmoid colon
O. rectum

O. is correct.
Cloaca develops into the rectum and the urinary bladder.

12.055 Which of the following structures is secondarily retroperitoneal AND NOT innervated by the vagus nerve?

A. liver
B. stomach
C. spleen
D. duodenum
E. pancreas
F. gall bladder
G. jejunum
H. ileum
I. cecum
J. appendix
K. ascending colon
L. transverse colon
M. descending colon
N. sigmoid colon
O. rectum

M. is correct.
The four GI structures that are secondarily retroperitoneal are: most of the duodenum, most of the pancreas, ascending colon and descending colon. All of these, except descending colon, are innervated by the parasympathetic fibers of the vagus nerve. Descending colon is innervated by branches of the pelvic splanchnic nerves from S2-4.

12.056 Normal gut rotation brings which structure to lie at McBurney's point?

A. liver
B. stomach
C. spleen
D. duodenum
E. pancreas
F. gall bladder
G. jejunum
H. ileum
I. cecum
J. appendix
K. ascending colon
L. transverse colon
M. descending colon
N. sigmoid colon
O. rectum

J. is correct.
McBurney's point, 1/3rd up along a line drawn between anterior superior iliac spine and umbilicus, is a fairly reliable landmark for the appendix. Variations is gut rotation, however, can cause the appendix to be located in other regions.

12.057 Which of the following structures is most closely related to the development both ventral and dorsal mesentery?

A. liver
B. stomach
C. spleen
D. duodenum
E. pancreas
F. gall bladder
G. jejunum
H. ileum
I. cecum
J. appendix
K. ascending colon
L. transverse colon
M. descending colon
N. sigmoid colon
O. rectum

B. is correct.
Ventral mesentery attaches dorsally to the stomach, and is also called ventral mesogastrium. The cranial part of the dorsal mesentery attaches to stomach and is called dorsal mesogastrium.

SECTION 13: UROGENITAL SYSTEM

13.001 Embryonic tissues or structures involved with uterine development include:

A. mesoderm
B. urogenital sinus
C. mesonephric ducts
D. endoderm

A. is correct.
The uterus is a derivative of the paramesonephric ducts which are of mesodermal origin. The urogenital sinus in the female develops into urinary bladder, urethra, lower vagina, urethral & paraurethral glands, greater vestibular glands & vestibule, but it does not develop into the uterus.

13.002 Structures derived from the mesonephric ducts include the:

A. seminiferous tubules
B. ureter
C. prostatic urethra
D. ductus deferens

D. is correct.
The mesonephric ducts in the male give rise to ductus epididymis, ductus deferens, ejaculatory ducts & seminal vesicles. Ureter, renal pelvis, renal calyces & renal collecting ducts arise from ureteric bud. Seminiferous tubules arise from the mesonephros. Prostatic urethra is a derivative of the urogenital sinus.

13.003 The scrotum of the male develops from:

A. endoderm of urogenital sinus
B. urethral groove
C. urogenital folds
D. genital swellings

D. is correct.
The urogenital folds are drawn out with the elongation of the phallus, forming the walls of the urogenital groove. The groove is lined with endoderm of the urogenital sinus. These folds close over the groove, forming the penile or spongy urethra. Genital swellings become scrotum or labia majora.

13.004 Horseshoe kidney:

A. involves splitting of the ureteric bud into a horseshoe shape
B. normally ascends to the L2 vertebral level
C. involves the persistence of the mesonephric kidney
D. results from fusion of the caudal poles of the kidneys

D. is correct.
Horseshoe kidney results from the fusion of the caudal poles of each kidney, forming one horseshoe-shaped structure. Its ascent is blocked by the inferior mesenteric artery at L3.

13.005 Which duct is NOT associated with urinary system development?

A. ureteric bud
B. paramesonephric duct
C. Wolffian duct
D. pronephric duct
E. mesonephric duct

B. is correct.
The paramesonephric duct arises along the urogenital ridge, separate from the urinary system. In the female, the paramesonephric duct develops into the uterine tubes, uterus and upper part of the vagina.

13.006 The penile urethra is derived from the:

A. urogenital sinus
B. pelvic part of the vesicourethral canal
C. phallic part of the vesicourethral canal
D. cloaca
E. mesonephric duct

A. is correct.
The penile urethra, all but navicular portion, develops from the urogenital sinus. The urogenital sinus also produces the urinary bladder, prostate and bulbourethral glands.

13.007 The structure dividing the cloaca into two parts is the:

A. distal retention band
B. transverse septum
C. urogenital sinus
D. urorectal septum
E. cloacal membrane

D. is correct.
The urorectal septum divides the cloaca into the urogenital sinus and the rectum, during the second month of development.

13.008 After the sinovaginal bulbs have proliferated and fused, they form a solid core of endodermal cells known as the:

A. sinus tubercle
B. prostatic utricle
C. vaginal plate
D. uterovaginal primordium
E. vault of the vagina

C. is correct.
The sinovaginal bulbs are evaginations from the urogenital sinus in the female. They proliferate, fuse, and form the vaginal plate, which then canalizes to form the lumen of vagina.

13.009 The layer of ectodermal cells which canalizes to form urethra at the distal end of the glans of the male phallus is known as the:

A. glandular plate
B. urethral plate
C. urogenital fold
D. primitive corpora spongiosum
E. phallic part of the UG sinus

A. is correct.
While most of the penile or spongy urethra arises from fusion of the urethral folds, the part of the urethra traversing the glans, or the glandular urethra, forms its lumen within a glandular plate formed from invaginating ectodermal cells.

13.010 The following structures are the derivatives of the primitive urogenital sinus EXCEPT:

A. most of the urinary bladder
B. male urethra
C. female urethra
D. upper part of vagina
E. vestibule of the vagina

D. is correct.
In the male, urogenital sinus gives rise to urinary bladder, all but the distal part of urethra, prostate and bulbourethral glands. In the female, it gives rise to urinary bladder, urethra, lower part of vagina, urethral & paraurethral glands, greater vestibular glands & vestibule. Upper vagina arises from paramesonephric ducts.

13.011 The following structures are developmental homologues:

A. scrotum - labia minora
B. gubernaculum testis/scrotal ligament - round ligament of uterus and ligament of ovary
C. ductus deferens - uterine tube
D. penile urethra - vagina

B. is correct.
The gubernaculum testis, round ligament of the uterus and ovarian ligament all develop from the gubernaculum. The prostatic urethra and vagina both develop from the urogenital sinus. Ductus deferens arises from mesonephric duct, while uterine tubes arise from the paramesonephric duct. Scrotum/labia majora are homologous.

13.012 The structures of the female pelvis representing the homologue of the gubernaculum testis are:

A. cardinal ligament of the uterus
B. round ligament of the uterus
C. suspensory ligament of the ovary
D. medial umbilical ligament

B. is correct.
Since the round ligament of the uterus and the ovarian ligament both arise from the gubernaculum, as does the scrotal ligament, they are homologous. Cardinal ligament is endopelvic fascia surrounding the uterine vessels, and it helps to support the uterus. Suspensory ligament of the ovary is peritoneum over ovarian vessels.

13.013 Which of the following ligaments is derived from peritoneum?

A. cardinal ligament of the uterus
B. puboprostatic ligament
C. ligament of the ovary
D. suspensory ligament of the ovary
E. round ligament of the uterus

D. is correct.
Suspensory ligament of the ovary is a fold of peritoneum overlying the ovarian vessels. Round ligament of the uterus and ligament of the ovary are remnants of the gubernaculum. Cardinal, uterosacral and puboprostatic ligaments are extraperitoneal connective tissue or endopelvic fascia. Broad ligament is also peritoneum.

13.014 The structures listed below are of mesodermal origin EXCEPT:

A. cortex of the kidney
B. renal pyramids
C. renal pelvis
D. ureter
E. urethra

E. is correct.
The urethra is an endodermal structure, having developed from the cloaca, by way of the urogenital sinus. Kidney cortex develops from the metanephric blastema, from mesoderm. Ureteric bud, from the mesonephros and therefore mesoderm, gives rise to the urinary ducts.

13.015 The embryonic origin(s) of the vagina is/are:

A. urethral folds
B. genital tubercle
C. genital swellings
D. sinovaginal bulbs
E. cloaca

D. is correct.
The cloaca is divided by the urorectal septum into the urogenital sinus and the rectum. The lower part of vagina then develops within the vaginal plate, which forms from endodermal outgrowths from the posterior wall of the urogenital sinus called sinovaginal bulbs.

13.016 The embryonic origin(s) of the labia minora is/are:

A. urethral folds
B. genital tubercle
C. genital swellings
D. sinovaginal bulbs
E. cloacal membrane

A. is correct.
The labia minora develop from the urethral or urogenital folds. In the male, the urethral folds ultimately fuse, forming the ventral aspect of the penis. The labia majora and the scrotum arise from the genital folds or swellings.

13.017 The embryonic origin(s) of the penile urethra is/are:

A. urethral folds
B. genital tubercle
C. genital swellings
D. sinovaginal bulbs
E. cloacal membrane

A. is correct.
The labia minora develop from the urethral or urogenital folds. In the male, the urethral folds ultimately fuse, enclosing the penile or spongy urethra. However, the urethra passing through the glans is formed by canalization of the glandular plate.

13.018 The embryonic origin(s) of the scrotum is/are:

A. urethral folds
B. genital tubercle
C. genital swellings
D. sinovaginal bulbs
E. cloacal membrane

C. is correct.
The scrotum in the male and the labia majora arise from the genital swellings or folds. Cloacal membrane is subdivided into the urorectal membrane and anal membrane by the urogenital septum. These membranes should rupture during the 9th week.

13.019 The urogenital sinus is derived from:
- A. the mesonephric or Wolffian ducts
- B. the paramesonephric or Mullerian ducts
- C. both
- D. neither

D. is correct.
The urogenital sinus is formed when the urorectal septum divides the cloaca into the urogenital sinus and rectum. Mesonephric ducts empty into urogenital sinus posteriorly, and paramesonephric ducts contact the posterior aspect of the sinus and induce the development of the vagina.

13.020 The uterine tubes are derived from:
- A. the mesonephric or Wolffian ducts
- B. the paramesonephric or Mullerian ducts
- C. both
- D. neither

B. is correct.
The uterine tubes, uterus and upper vagina develop from the female genital ducts, the paramesonephric ducts. Mesonephric duct becomes the epididymis, ductus deferens, seminal vesical and ejaculatory duct in the male. Female remnants of mesonephric duct may include epoophoron, paroophoron and Gartner's duct cysts.

13.021 The seminal vesicles are derived from:
- A. the mesonephric or Wolffian ducts
- B. the paramesonephric or Mullerian ducts
- C. both
- D. neither

A. is correct.
The male seminal vesicles are derived from the male genital ducts, the mesonephric ducts. The male remnant of the paramesonephric ducts is the prostatic utricle, a small, blind pouch located in the seminal colliculus within the prostatic urethra, near the orifices of the ejaculatory ducts.

13.022 The appendix of the epididymis is derived from:
- A. the mesonephric or Wolffian ducts
- B. the paramesonephric or Mullerian ducts
- C. both
- D. neither

A. is correct.
The appendix of the epididymis is a worthless, vestigial appendage on the head of the epididymis that is derived from the mesonephric ducts. The only thing that it is known to do is show up on National Board exams. The appendix of the testis, equally worthless, is a vestige of the paramesonephric duct.

13.023 Which of the following definitions is NOT true:
- A. hypospadias - defect in the wall of the male urethra
- B. cryptorchismus - failure of descent of the testis
- C. true hermaphrodite has male and female gonads
- D. hydrocele testis - collection of fluid within the testis tubules

D. is correct.
Hypospadias results from incomplete fusion of the urogenital folds ventrally. Failure of testes descent is cryptorchismus, which can result in sterility or predilection to testicular cancer. A true hermaphrodite has gonads of both sexes. Hydrocele testis is an accumulation of fluid in tunica vaginalis testis.

13.024 With regard to the development of the testis:
- A. The embryonic origin of the germ cells is from the germinal epithelium of the gonad.
- B. Ductuli efferentes of the testis are derived from mesonephric tubules.
- C. The testis descends through the inguinal canal due to contraction of the gubernaculum.
- D. The duct of the epididymis, if uncoiled, would measure less than a foot in length.

B. is correct.
The origin of germ cells is the yolk sac endoderm. The efferent ductules are derived from mesonephric tubules. The testes descend because the gubernaculum fails to elongate as rapidly as the body, and possibly also due to some contraction of gubernaculum. Strange but true: the duct of the epididymis is 15-20 feet uncoiled.

13.025 The uterus arises from:

A. endoderm
B. mesoderm
C. both
D. neither

B. is correct.
The uterus arises from the paramesonephric ducts, mesodermal tissue from the urogenital ridge, which is intermediate mesoderm.

13.026 The vagina arises from:

A. endoderm
B. mesoderm
C. both
D. neither

C. is correct.
The upper one-third of the vagina develops from the paramesonephric ducts, which are mesodermal. The lower 2/3rds of the vagina develops from the urogenital sinus & sinovaginal bulbs, which are endodermal.

13.027 The calyces of the kidney arise from:

A. endoderm
B. mesoderm
C. both
D. neither

B. is correct.
The calyces of the kidney develop from the ureteric bud, which comes off of the mesonephric duct. The mesonephric duct, ureteric bud and the metanephric blastema are mesodermal.

13.028 The following statements are true with respect to the development of the urogenital system:

A. The germ cells, ova and sperm cells, are derived from the intermediate mesoderm.
B. The epididymis is derived from the mesonephric duct.
C. The Wolffian duct always disappears without a trace in the female.
D. The urinary bladder in the male is of endodermal origin only.

B. is correct.
Germ cells are derived from yolk sac endoderm. Epididymis forms from the mesonephric duct. The Wolffian or mesonephric duct may persist in the female as epoophoron & paroophoron near ovary, or as Gartner's duct cysts. Bladder is from the endodermal UG sinus, but bladder trigone is from the mesodermal mesonephric ducts.

13.029 The following structures are directly or indirectly derived from the mesonephric or Wolffian duct EXCEPT:

A. part of the epididymis
B. part of the kidney
C. part of the urinary bladder
D. seminal vesicles
E. prostate

E. is correct.
The prostate is derived from the urogenital sinus, with no contribution from the mesonephric ducts. Ureteric bud, from mesonephric duct, gives rise to the collecting system of the kidney. A portion of mesonephric ducts becomes incorporated into the trigone region of the bladder. Seminal vesicles bud from the mesonephric duct.

13.030 The following structures are the derivatives of the primitive urogenital sinus EXCEPT:

A. most of the urinary bladder
B. male urethra
C. female urethra
D. lower vagina
E. ejaculatory ducts

E. is correct.
The ejaculatory ducts are derivatives of the mesonephric ducts. All of the others have at least some contribution from the urogenital sinus.

13.031 Which of the following is NOT a correct association:

A. congenital polycystic kidney - result of defective union of mesonephric and metanephric units
B. urachal fistula - persistence of allantoic duct
C. double ureter - early splitting of the ureteric bud
D. hydrocele testis - accumulation of fluid within the testis

D. is correct.
Congenital polycystic kidney occurs when the collecting system and the cortex of kidney fail to unite correctly. A urachal fistula results from persistent allantoic duct. Splitting of the ureteric bud can cause double ureter. Hydrocele is accumulation of fluid in the tunica vaginalis testis, not testis itself.

13.032 The embryonic origin of tubuli recti of the kidney is:

A. mesonephric tubules
B. Wolffian duct
C. ureteric bud or metanephric diverticulum
D. metanephric blastema
E. metanephric glomeruli

C. is correct.
The tubuli recti of the kidney are part of the collecting system, rather than the excretory system of the kidney. Therefore, they are derived from the ureteric bud. The excretory system of kidney, the cortex, develops from the metanephric blastema.

13.033 The derivatives of the Wolffian duct include each of the following EXCEPT:

A. longitudinal duct of Gartner
B. round ligament of uterus
C. ductus deferens
D. duct of the epididymis
E. ejaculatory duct

B. is correct.
Gartner's duct, like the appendix of the epididymis, holds more importance to National Board examiners than anyone else. It is a vestigial remnant of the mesonephric duct in the female. The round ligament of the uterus is derived from the gubernaculum, rather than the mesonephric duct.

13.034 Of the following, the one most closely associated with the prostate gland is:

A. mesonephric tubules
B. mesonephric duct
C. paramesonephric duct
D. genital swellings
E. urogenital sinus

E. is correct.
In the male, the urogenital sinus gives rise to the urinary bladder, all but distal urethra, prostate and bulbourethral glands. In the female, it gives rise to the urinary bladder, urethra, lower part of vagina, vestibule, urethral and paraurethral glands and greater vestibular glands.

13.035 Of the following, the one most closely associated with the oviduct is:

A. mesonephric tubules
B. mesonephric duct
C. paramesonephric duct
D. genital swellings
E. urogenital sinus

C. is correct.
Paramesonephric ducts give rise to the oviducts or uterine tubes, uterus and upper portion of the vagina. In males, the prostatic utricle and the appendix of the testis are vestigial remnants of the paramesonephric ducts.

13.036 Of the following, the one most closely associated with the efferent ducts of the testes is:

A. mesonephric tubules
B. mesonephric duct
C. paramesonephric duct
D. genital swellings
E. urogenital sinus

A. is correct.
The efferent ductules of the testes are the only functional derivatives of the mesonephric tubules.

13.037 Of the following, the one most closely associated with the vestibule in the female is:

A. mesonephric tubules
B. mesonephric duct
C. paramesonephric duct
D. genital swellings
E. urogenital sinus

E. is correct.
In the male, the urogenital sinus gives rise to the urinary bladder, all but distal urethra, prostate and bulbourethral glands. In the female, it gives rise to the urinary bladder, urethra, lower part of vagina, vestibule, urethral and paraurethral glands and greater vestibular glands.

13.038 Of the following, the one most closely associated with the seminal vesicle is:

A. mesonephric tubules
B. mesonephric duct
C. paramesonephric duct
D. genital swellings
E. urogenital sinus

B. is correct.
In addition to its urinary contributions in each sex, the mesonephric duct gives rise to the ductus epididymis, ductus deferens, ejaculatory duct and seminal vesicle in the male.

13.039 Of the following, the one most closely associated with the urethra in the female is:

A. mesonephric tubules
B. mesonephric duct
C. paramesonephric duct
D. genital swellings
E. urogenital sinus

E. is correct.
In the male, the urogenital sinus gives rise to the urinary bladder, prostate, bulbourethral glands and all but distal urethra. In the female, it gives rise to the urinary bladder, urethra, lower part of vagina, vestibule, urethral and paraurethral glands and greater vestibular glands.

13.040 Which of the following is NOT true concerning urinary system development:

A. the epithelium of the male and female urethra is of endodermal origin
B. the distal convoluted tubules arise from the metanephric blastema
C. the collecting ducts arise from the ureteric bud
D. the glomerulus arises from the mesonephric duct

D. is correct.
The urethra in both sexes is from the urogenital sinus, which is from the cloaca, an endodermal structure. The kidney arises from two sources. Metanephric blastemata end in distal convoluted tubules which join the collecting ducts from the ureteric bud. The glomerulus is a vascular structure, not mesonephric.

13.041 In the urinary system:

A. pressence of feces at the umbilicus of an infant may be indicative of urachal fistula
B. renal agenesis is most likely due to an endocrine imbalance
C. urine is excreted into the amniotic fluid during the second half of pregnancy
D. congenital polycystic kidney is most likely due to a blockage of the urethra

C. is correct.
Urachal fistula is persistence of allantoic duct from umbilicus to bladder. Renal agenesis is not caused by endocrine imbalance. Lack of urine excretion into the amniotic fluid during 2nd half of pregnancy reduces amniotic fluid causing oligohydramnios. Abnormal metanephric and ureteric union causes polycystic kidney.

13.042 The urinary system in the human does NOT:

A. develop from intermediate mesoderm
B. develop from two different sources
C. develop in close association with the genital system
D. have a functional pronephros during the 4th week of gestation

D. is correct.
Both urinary and genital systems develop largely from intermediate mesoderm. The urinary system has 2 sources: metanephric blastemata and ureteric buds. The pronephros is a nonfunctional forerunner of the urinary system that disappears by the end of the 4th week.

13.043 Exstrophy of the bladder:

A. is frequently accompanied by hypospadias
B. is due to a primary defect in endoderm migration
C. is due to a deficient growth of the urorectal septum
D. exposes the posterior wall of the bladder to the outside

D. is correct.
Exstrophy of the bladder involves rupture or underdevelopment of the anterior abdominal wall, causing the posterior wall of bladder to be exposed. It may be caused by failure of mesenchyme migration to form the anterior abdominal wall as well as the anterior wall of the bladder. It is often accompanied by epispadias.

13.044 A true hermaphrodite can be distinguished from a pseudohermaphrodite by:

A. chromosome complement
B. behavior
C. appearance of external genitalia
D. presence of both testicular and ovarian tissue

D. is correct.
The characteristic of true hermaphrodism is the presence of gonads of each sex. True hermaphrodism is extremely rare.

13.045 Abnormal development of external genitalia in an XY male would NOT be due to:

A. 5-alpha reductase deficiency
B. androgen receptor deficiency
C. failure of androgen-receptor complex to elicit a response in the nucleus
D. failure in the cellular conversion of testosterone to estradiol

D. is correct.
Abnormal development of external genitalia in an XY male can be caused by 5-alpha reductase deficiency, a deficiency in androgen receptors, or the inability of the androgen-receptor complex to elicit a nuclear response.

13.046 In the absence of an inducing substance from the gonad of an XY fetus:

A. the indifferent external genitalia may develop into female or male structures
B. a true hermaphrodite develops
C. derivatives of the paramesonephric duct may persist
D. the indifferent stage in the genital system persists in postnatal life

C. is correct.
In the absence of androgens and Mullerian inhibiting substance in the XY fetus, maternal and placental estrogens are cause female external genitalia and the persistent paramesonephric duct to develop. A true hermaphrodite requires gonads of each sex, and the indifferent gonad stage does not persist.

13.047 In the development of the genital system:

A. primordial germ cells induce the indifferent gonad to develop into ovary or testis
B. primitive sex cords arise from coelomic epithelium of the genital ridge in embryos of both sexes
C. cortical cords give rise to follicular cells
D. medullary cords give rise to seminiferous tubules in the male
E. all of the above are correct

E. is correct.
Primordial germ cells determine the route of differentiation of the indifferent gonad. Germ cells migrate from the yolk sac to genital ridge, where they form primitive sex cords. A Y chromosome causes the cords to form medullary cords that become seminiferous tubules. Without Y, cortical cords form and become follicular cells.

13.048 An individual has 44 + XY chromosomes with testes but his tissues are unresponsive to androgens. This individual may have:

A. uterine tubes
B. blind ending vagina
C. prostate gland
D. external appearance of a male

B. is correct.
In this individual, presence of Mullerian inhibiting substance would still cause regression of the paramesonephric ducts. However, the absence of androgen sensitivity prevents the development of male external genitalia, and maternal and placental estrogens induce development of female genitalia.

13.049 In the urinary system:

A. the excretory units are outgrowths from collecting ducts
B. the bladder is a derivative of the urogenital sinus
C. the collecting ducts are derived from the metanephric blastema
D. a urachal fistula is a remnant of the cloaca

B. is correct.
Collecting system, collecting ducts to ureter, arise from ureteric bud. Excretory units, Bowman's capsule to distal convoluted tubule, arise from metanephric blastema. Bladder is from urogenital sinus. Allantois, becoming urachus, connects bladder to umbilicus. If it persists, urine leaks at umbilicus via a urachal fistula.

13.050 In the human, the mesonephros:

A. is important in development of the internal genital organs in the female
B. is the definitive unit of the kidney
C. contributes to the outlet ducts from the testis
D. has a dual origin from splanchnic mesoderm

C. is correct.
The mesonephros is the male genital duct system precursor. It does not contribute significantly to female genital development. The mesonephros forms excretory units which regress to be replaced by the definitive kidney, the metanephros. Kidney & gonad development occurs within the intermediate mesoderm.

13.051 In the genital system:

A duplication abnormalities of the uterus may be due to lack of fusion of paramesonephric ducts
B. the most common cause of female pseudohermaphroditism is excessive androgen production
C. cryptorchism may be due to abnormal androgen production
D. pure gonadal dysgenesis may be due to failure of primordial germ cells to seed the indifferent gonad
E. all of the above are correct

E. is correct.
A bicornuate uterus and double uterus results from incomplete fusion of the paramesonephric ducts. Too much androgen in females causes pseudohermaphrodism; too little in males may cause cryptorchism. If the germ cells never hit their mark, they cannot induce gonad formation.

13.052 Which of the following associations are correct?

A. renal pelvis - ureteric bud
B. ureter - ureteric bud
C. urethra - urogenital sinus
D. median umbilical ligament - urachus
E. all of the above are correct

E. is correct.
Ureteric bud gives rise to everything from collecting ducts through ureter. Derivatives of UG sinus include bladder & urethra of both sexes, prostate & bulbourethral glands, lower vagina and urethral, paraurethral & vestibular glands. Allantois becomes urachus, which then becomes median umbilical ligament.

13.053 Bilateral renal agenesis:

A. is due to an endocrine imbalance
B. is incompatible with life
C. results when the kidneys fail to migrate out of the pelvis
D. is due to the absence of a paramesonephric duct

B. is correct.
You can't live without any kidneys. The agenesis is not due to a failure of kidney migration, but to an early degeneration of the ureteric bud or to a lack of induction of the metanephric mesoderm by ureteric bud. Oligohydramnios, or very little amniotic fluid, would result, since fetal urine adds to amniotic fluid.

13.054 In the female:

A. the clitoris forms from the genital swellings
B. the ureter forms from the urogenital sinus
C. the urogenital groove remains open and forms the vestibule
D. the labia minora are homologous to the scrotum

C. is correct.
Genital tubercle forms the clitoris or glans of penis, making these homologous structures. Ureter is from ureteric bud. Urogenital groove closes on the ventral surface of penis. In the female, it remains open to form vestibule. Scrotum & labia majora are also homologues, both from genital swellings.

13.055 In the development of the genital system, which is NOT correct:

A. a true hermaphrodite has testicular and ovarian tissue, regardless of genetic or phenotypic sex
B. genetic males convert testosterone to DHT, leading to the development of male external genitalia
C. testosterone is converted to estradiol in the brain, resulting in imprinting as male
D. the genetic sex always determines the development of the internal and external genitalia

D. is correct.
A true hermaphrodite has gonads of both sexes. Testosterone is converted to DHT, inducing development of male external genitalia, and estradiol in the brain, leading to male imprinting. As is seen in certain defects, genetic sex does not always lead to proper genital development.

13.056 In the male, which is NOT correct:

A. elongation of the genital tubercle forms the phallus
B. fusion of the urethral folds establishes the penile urethra
C. the genital swellings form the scrotum
D. abnormal positioning of the genital tubercle causes hypospadias

D. is correct.
Genital tubercle elongates to form phallus. On its ventral surface, the urethral/genital folds fuse to enclose penile urethra. In the male, genital swellings also fuse to form scrotum. Hypospadias results from failure of urethral fold fusion, leaving a ventral slit in the penis.

13.057 Concerning testicular feminization syndrome, which is NOT correct:

A. individuals are males with a 44XY chromosome complement
B. the paramesonephric system is suppressed, oviducts and uterus are absent
C. external genital tissue is unresponsive to androgen and develops along female lines
D. there is a lack of androgen production by the testes

D. is correct.
In testicular feminization, testes in the genotypic male do their job. They produce plenty of androgens and MIS, but the peripheral tissues are insensitive to androgens. Even though MIS causes the paramesonephric system to regress, the external genitalia still develop along female lines.

13.058 At about what age do the testes begin to descend into the scrotum?

A. 4 months
B. 5 months
C. 6 months
D. 7 months
E. 8 months

E. is correct.
The testes begin to descend around the 3rd month. This is due to differential growth of the body compared to the gubernaculum testis, which attaches testis to genital swelling. Testes descend to the inguinal region, but do not enter scrotum until shortly before birth, or roughly 8th month.

13.059 Which of the following are derivatives of the human pronephros?

A. renal capsule
B. Bowman's capsule
C. both
D. neither

D. is correct.
The human pronephros forms and degenerates so quickly that nothing at all really comes from it.

13.060 Which of the following are functional derivatives of the mesonephros?

A. efferent ductules of the male
B. fallopian tube of the female
C. both
D. neither

A. is correct.
The efferent ductules in the male are derivatives of the mesonephric duct. The oviduct or fallopian or uterine tube of the female is of paramesonephric origin.

13.061 Embryologically, each uriniferous tubule consists of two parts which become confluent at the junction of the:

A. ascending limb of Henle's loop and the distal convoluted tubule
B. renal corpuscle and the proximal convoluted tubule
C. descending and ascending limbs of the loop of Henle
D. proximal convoluted tubule and the loop of Henle
E. distal convoluted tubule and the collecting tubule

E. is correct.
Everything from Bowman's capsule to the distal convoluted tubule develops from the metanephric cap. Everything from the collecting tubules through the ureter develops from the ureteric bud. Therefore the junction between the two occurs between the distal convoluted tubule and the collecting tubule.

13.062 The ureteric bud appears as an outgrowth from the:

A. metanephric mass
B. lateral plate mesoderm
C. urogenital sinus
D. allantoic duct
E. mesonephric duct

E. is correct.
The ureteric bud is an outgrowth of the mesonephric duct. It forms the ureter, renal pelvis, calyces and collecting ducts.

13.063 The paramesonephric ducts in female embryos give rise to the:

A. uterine tubes and uterus
B. epoophoron
C. inferior fifth of the vagina
D. round ligament of the uterus
E. ovarian ligament

A. is correct.
The paramesonephric ducts in the female develop into the uterine tubes, the uterus and the upper 1/3 of the vagina. The epoophoron come from the mesonephric tubules. The lower portion of the vagina develops from the urogenital sinus. The round ligament and the ovarian ligament are from the gubernaculum.

13.064 Which of the following gives rise to the labia majora?

A. genital folds
B. genital swellings
C. genital tubercle
D. urorectal fold
E. inguinal fold

B. is correct.
Labia majora arise from the genital swellings. Their counterpart in the male is the scrotum, which also arises from the genital swellings. The genital tubercle forms the distal end of penis and most of clitoris.

13.065 Which of the following is a remnant of the gubernaculum?

A. prostatic utricle
B. ductus deferens
C. median umbilical ligament
D. vagina
E. labium majora
F. seminal vesicle
G. proper ovarian ligament
H. urinary bladder
I. clitoris
J. ureter
K. uterine tube
L. testis
M. kidney
N. labium minora

G. is correct.
In response to male hormones, the gubernaculum shortens to draw the testis into the scrotum. It becomes the scrotal ligament, anchoring the testis within the scrotum. In the female, gubernaculum becomes the round ligament of the uterus and the proper ovarian ligament.

13.066 Which of the following is a remnant of the allantois?

A. prostatic utricle
B. ductus deferens
C. median umbilical ligament
D. vagina
E. labium majora
F. seminal vesicle
G. proper ovarian ligament
H. urinary bladder
I. clitoris
J. ureter
K. uterine tube
L. testis
M. kidney
N. labium minora

C. is correct.
The allantois disappears, becoming the urachus. The median umbilical ligament is the adult remnant of the urachus. Urachal cysts or fistulae result from incomplete disappearance of the urachus.

13.067 Which of the following develops from the intermediate mesoderm in response to induction by the ureteric bud ?

A. prostatic utricle
B. ductus deferens
C. median umbilical ligament
D. vagina
E. labium majora
F. seminal vesicle
G. proper ovarian ligament
H. urinary bladder
I. clitoris
J. ureter
K. uterine tube
L. testis
M. kidney
N. labium minora

M. is correct.
Testis and kidney both develop from intermediate mesoderm. However, testis develops from the mesonephros, and mesonephric duct becomes ductus deferens. Ureteric bud grows from the mesonephric duct into the metanephric blastema, inducing it to form the kidney.

13.068 Which of the following develops from the genital tubercle?

A. prostatic utricle
B. ductus deferens
C. median umbilical ligament
D. vagina
E. labium majora
F. seminal vesicle
G. proper ovarian ligament
H. urinary bladder
I. clitoris
J. ureter
K. uterine tube
L. testis
M. kidney
N. labium minora

I. is correct.
The genital tubercle becomes clitoris or distal penis.

SECTION 14: NERVOUS SYSTEM, EYE AND EAR

14.001 Which structures are derived from the optic cup?

A. neural retina
B. iris epithelium
C. pigment layer of the retina
D. ciliary body epithelium
E. all of the above are correct

E. is correct.
The optic cup ultimately develops into the pigment layer of the retina, the neural retina, the epithelium of the iris and the epithelium of the ciliary body.

14.002 The optic nerve is derived from what embryonic tissue?

A. neural crest
B. head mesenchyme
C. endoderm
D. mesoderm
E. ectoderm

E. is correct.
The optic nerve is derived from nervous tissue, therefore ectoderm, but not neural crest. Optic sulci of the neural folds forming the forebrain send out the optic vesicles, which then develop into the optic cups connected to forebrain by the optic stalk. The optic stalk becomes the optic nerve.

14.003 Which portion of the ear is derived from endoderm?

A. semicircular canals
B. tympanic cavity
C. external auditory meatus
D. bony labyrinth
E. cochlea

B. is correct.
The tympanic cavity is endodermal in origin, derived from the 1st pharyngeal pouch. The internal ear, including the cochlea, bony labyrinth and semicircular canals, are derived from the ectodermal otic placode. External auditory meatus, from 1st pharyngeal cleft, is also ectodermal.

14.004 The otic vesicle does NOT develop into the:

A. membranous cochlea
B. endolymphatic duct
C. saccule
D. otic placode

D. is correct.
Otic vesicle develops into the saccule, cochlear duct or membranous cochlea, utricle, semicircular canals and endolymphatic duct & sac. It develops FROM the ectodermal otic placode.

14.005 Which of the following structures is derived from mesoderm?

A. optic nerve
B. retina
C. iris epithelium
D. superior oblique muscle

D. is correct.
The optic nerve, retina and iris epithelium arise from the optic vesicle, an evagination of the forebrain. Since forebrain is nervous tissue, it is ectodermal. The superior oblique muscle is a muscle, so it is mesodermal in origin, somitomeric mesoderm, in particular.

14.006 Neural crest cells differentiate into:

A. postganglionic sympathetic cell bodies
B. cells of the inferior mesenteric ganglion
C. adrenal medullary cells
D. cells of the enteric plexus
E. all of the above are correct

E. is correct.
Neural crest cells give rise to the peripheral parts of the autonomic nervous system, which includes all sympathetic and parasympathetic ganglia. Neural crest cells form all sensory ganglia of the peripheral nervous system. Neural crest cells also populate the adrenal medulla.

14.007 The ganglia of the autonomic nervous system are derived from:

A. ectoderm
B. endoderm
C. both
D. neither

A. is correct.
The ganglia of the autonomic nervous system are of neural crest origin. They are therefore ectodermal, as is the entire nervous system.

14.008 Of the following, the item most closely associated with the regulation of visceral and endocrine functions is:

A. telencephalon
B. diencephalon
C. mesencephalon
D. metencephalon
E. myelencephalon

B. is correct.
The hypothalamus of the diencephalon is the control center for visceral and endocrine functions.

14.009 Of the following, the item most closely associated with the pons is:

A. telencephalon
B. diencephalon
C. mesencephalon
D. metencephalon
E. myelencephalon

D. is correct.
The metencephalon differentiates into the cerebellum, the coordination center for posture and movement and the pons, which serves as a neural relay center.

14.010 Of the following, the item most closely associated with visual reflexes is:

A. telencephalon
B. diencephalon
C. mesencephalon
D. metencephalon
E. myelencephalon

C. is correct.
The superior colliculi of the mesencephalon serve as reflex centers for visual input.

14.011 Of the following, the one most closely associated with the cerebrum is:

A. telencephalon
B. diencephalon
C. mesencephalon
D. metencephalon
E. myelencephalon

A. is correct.
The cerebrum arises from the telencephalon. Telencephalon, the most rostral part of the brain vesicles, develops from the prosencephalon as lateral outgrowths, the cerebral hemispheres and an intermediate area, the lamina terminalis. Lamina terminalis develops into the commissures connecting the hemispheres.

14.012 Of the following, the one most closely associated with the 3rd ventricle is:

A. telencephalon
B. diencephalon
C. mesencephalon
D. metencephalon
E. myelencephalon

B. is correct.
The 3rd ventricle lies within the thalamic area in the diencephalon. The lateral ventricles are cavities of the forebrain cerebral vesicles, from telencephalon. The 4th ventricle lies within the metencephalon.

14.013 Myelomeningocele is often associated with a caudal displacement of medulla and a portion of the cerebellum into the vertebral canal.

A. true
B. false

A. is correct.
Myelomeningocele in which both nervous tissue and meningeal tissue herniate through a cleft in the spinal column is called the Arnold-Chiari syndrome. The herniation blocks cerebrospinal fluid flow from the 4th ventricle and produces hydrocephaly.

14.014 The sympathetic nervous system is derived mostly from neural crest cells.

A. true
B. false

A. is correct.
Neural crest cells give rise to dorsal root ganglia and neurons, the peripheral ganglia of the sympathetic & parasympathetic nervous systems, odontoblasts, meninges, mesenchyme of the head & neck, Schwann cells, adrenal medulla and pigment cells of the skin.

14.015 Spina bifida occulta and encephalomeningocele result from a defect in neural tube closure.

A. true
B. false

B. is correct.
These malformations result from a defect in the skeletal system, not neural tube closure. Spina bifida occulta is a defect of the neural arch of the vertebral column. Meningoencephalocele is a herniation of meninges and part of the brain through a defect in the calvaria or skull cap.

14.016 Microglial cells arise from gliablasts after the production of neuroblasts has ceased.

A. true
B. false

B. is correct.
Microglial cells do not arise from gliablasts. They arise from mesenchyme cells.

14.017 Anencephaly is more frequent in females than males.

A. true
B. false

A. is correct.
Anencephaly, a failure of the neural tube to close at the cephalic end, is more common in females than males and is more common in whites than in blacks.

14.018 During maturation of the nervous system:

A. fiber tracts appear to become myelinated about the time they start to function
B. all myelination of nerve fibers is by oligodendroglial cells
C. the first reflexes appear in the caudal region
D. there is no movement of the embryo/fetus until the 15th week

A. is correct.
Fiber tracts appear to become myelinated about the time that they start to function. Myelination is carried out centrally by oligodendroglia and peripherally by Schwann cells. Movements in the fetus usually begin toward the end of the third month, but are not readily felt by the mother until the 5th month.

14.019 Cerebrospinal fluid:

A. is produced in choroid plexuses
B. circulates in the ventricular system of the brain and in the subarachnoid spaces
C. re-enters the venous blood at the arachnoid granulations
D. blockage of its circulation can lead to internal or external hydrocephalus
E. all of the above are correct

E. is correct.
Cerebrospinal fluid is produced by ependymal cells of the choroid plexus. It circulates within the ventricles of the brain, the central canal of the spinal cord and the subarachnoid space. It is resorbed into the venous system via arachnoid granulations. If flow is blocked, CSF accumulates & creates hydrocephalus.

14.020 In the development of the nervous system:
A. there are five primary brain vesicles
B. during the 5th week, each brain vesicle subdivides into 2 parts
C. the pontine flexure is in a direction opposite the mesencephalic and cervical flexure
D. neural epithelial cells are found in the marginal layer

C. is correct.
There are initially 3 brain vesicles: prosencephalon, mesencephalon & rhombencephalon. The pros- & rhombencephalon divide into 2 parts. The pontine flexure is opposite to the mesencephalic and cervical flexures. The marginal layer contains the nerve fibers arising from the neuroblasts.

14.021 In the development of the nervous system:
A. the sulcus limitans is found in the diencephalon
B. the infundibulum is an outgrowth of the telencephalon that develops into the neurohypophysis
C. sensory nuclei in the hindbrain lie ventral to the sulcus limitans
D. the inner ear is derived from surface ectoderm

D. is correct.
The sulcus limitans is a lateral, longitudinal groove dividing basal and alar plates. The infundibulum is an outpouching of the hypothalamic region that becomes neurohypophysis. Sensory nuclei lie dorsal to the sulcus limitans. Internal ear is from thickened surface ectoderm (otic placode) near rhombencephalon.

14.022 In the development of the nervous system:
A. the neural groove forms from the neural plate
B. the neural folds are composed of neuroepithelial cells
C. the neural tube maintains temporary contact with the amniotic cavity via neuropores
D. neuroepithelial cells give rise to both neuroblasts and gliablasts
E. all of the above are correct

E. is correct.
The neural groove forms from the neural plate when lateral parts of the plate elevate to form neural folds. Neural folds are composed of neuroepithelium which gives rise to neuroblasts, gliablasts & ependymal cells. After the neural tube forms, it maintains contact with the amniotic cavity via cranial & caudal neuropores.

14.023 Identify the correct association(s):
A. basal plate - sensory neurons
B. mantle layer - neuroblasts
C. marginal layer - gray matter
D. alar plate - choroid plexus

B. is correct.
The sensory neurons lie in the alar plate. The neuroblasts are in the mantle area. The marginal layer contains the white, myelinated nerve fibers. The choroid plexus is in the roof plate.

14.024 With respect to the nervous system, which of the following is NOT correct:
A. a muscle's nerve supply can be used as an indicator of its level of origin and path of migration
B. Rathke's pouch is an outgrowth of oral ectoderm that becomes the anterior lobe of the hypophysis
C. the sulcus limitans marks the boundary between motor and sensory areas
D. sensory nuclei in the hindbrain lie ventral to motor nuclei

D. is correct.
The nerve supply travels with the muscle, indicating its origin and migration path. Rathke's pouch, from which the anterior pituitary is formed, is from oral ectoderm. Sulcus limitans divides motor and sensory areas. Sensory nuclei in the hindbrain lie dorsal to the motor nuclei.

14.025 In the list below, which embryonic structures are correctly matched with the adult structure and function?

A. mesencephalon - colliculi - visual and auditory reflexes
B. metencephalon - medulla - reflex center
C. telencephalon - thalamus - sensory relay and integration
D. telencephalon - cerebellum - motor coordination

A. is correct.
The colliculi serve as relays for auditory and visual reflexes and arise from the mesencephalon. The medulla is derived from myelencephalon. The diencephalon contains the thalamus, a sensory relay station. The cerebellum arises from metencephalon.

14.026 Myelination:

A. is accomplished by neurilemma or Schwann cells in peripheral nerves
B. is accomplished by oligodendroglial cells within the spinal cord
C. continues after birth
D. is related to function
E. all of the above are correct

E. is correct.
Schwann cells do the myelination peripherally, while oligodendroglia cells do it centrally. Myelination continues for a year postnatally. The myelin coating is extremely important to nerve conduction velocity along the nerve.

14.027 Hydrocephalus:

A. exhibits decreased accumulation of CSF within the ventricles or between the brain and dura mater
B. is accompanied by an excessive amount of amniotic fluid
C. may be caused by an obstruction of the aqueduct of Sylvius
D. may be caused by an absence of the choroid plexuses

C. is correct.
An excessive accumulation of CSF within the ventricular system is called hydrocephalus. This is often caused by obstruction of the aqueduct of Sylvius. It is unrelated to the amount of amniotic fluid, and an absence of the choroid plexuses, which form the CSF, would lead to a scarcity of CSF.

14.028 Spina bifida cystica and meningoencephalocele:

A. are often caused by a failure of the neural tube to close
B. have their inception during the fourth week of development
C. always occur together in the affected individual
D. have as their primary cause a defect in development of bone

D. is correct.
Spina bifida cystica and cranial meningoencephalocele arise due to a failure in bone development, not neural tube development. Neural tube defects, like rachischisis and anencephaly, result from failure of the neural folds to fuse during the 4th week. Bone surrounding the neural tube forms later than the CNS.

14.029 Meningoencephalocele:

A. is due to the failure of the neural tube to close
B. is often associated with displacement of medulla and some cerebellum into the vertebral canal
C. most frequently is located in the cervical cord region
D. is not related to hydrocephaly

B. is correct.
Meningoencephalocele results from defective skull formation. It is often seen in conjunction with hydrocephaly and caudal displacement of the medulla and part of the cerebellum. This group of defects is called the Arnold-Chiari syndrome.

14.030 Anencephaly:

A. is the result of failure of the cephalic part of the neural tube to form
B. has its inception during the 5th week of development
C. is seen more frequently in females than in males
D. is accompanied by a deficiency in amniotic fluid

C. is correct.
Anencephaly occurs when the cephalic part of the neural tube fails to close. The reflex to swallow amniotic fluid does not develop and excess amniotic fluid, or polyhydramnios, results. It is 4 times more common in females than in males. Neural tube forms from the fusion of neural folds during the 4th week.

14.031 Congenital absence of neural crest cells could result in:

A. absence of sympathetic chain ganglia
B. facial malformations
C. absence of adrenal medulla
D. absence of pigment cells
E. all of the above are correct

E. is correct.
Neural crest cells form all sensory and autonomic ganglia, Schwann cells, meninges of the brain & spinal cord, adrenal medulla, pigment cells of the skin and connective tissues of the head and neck, including odontoblasts for dentin of the teeth.

14.032 Which of the following is usually associated with anencephaly?

A. macrocephalus
B. hydrocephalus
C. cranioschisis
D. microcephalus
E. conical cranium

C. is correct.
Rachischisis is the failure of the neural tube to close, and when it occurs in the cranial region, it is referred to as cranioschisis. Cranioschisis means split skull.

14.033 The metencephalon forms the:

A. cerebellum
B. medulla oblongata
C. both
D. neither

A. is correct.
The metencephalon forms the cerebellum and pons. The medulla arises from the myelencephalon.

14.034 The mesencephalon differentiates into the:

A. cerebellum
B. pons
C. both
D. neither

D. is correct.
The cerebellum and pons are from the metencephalon. Mesencephalon or midbrain becomes the cerebral peduncles and the superior and inferior colliculi, and contains the cerebral aqueduct.

14.035 The brain flexure which develops between the metencephalon and the myelencephalon is called the:

A. pontine
B. hindbrain
C. cervical
D. cephalic
E. midbrain

A. is correct.
The pontine flexure occurs between the metencephalon, which forms the pons and cerebellum, and the myelencephalon, which forms the medulla. The two other flexures, the cephalic and the cervical, flex in a direction opposite that of the pontine.

14.036 The lateral longitudinal groove in the inner surface of the developing spinal cord is the:

A. neural groove
B. cuneate groove
C. sulcus limitans
D. longitudinal groove
E. transverse fold

C. is correct.
The sulcus limitans is the lateral groove of the developing spinal cord that separates the basal and alar plates. The basal plate goes on to become the ventral motor horn, and the alar plate goes on to become the dorsal sensory horn of the spinal cord.

14.037 At birth, the caudal end of the spinal cord lies at which vertebral level?

A. third sacral
B. first sacral
C. third lumbar
D. first lumbar
E. twelfth thoracic

C. is correct.
Early on, the spinal cord runs the entire length of the embryo, but because the rest of the body grows faster than the cord, it shortens in relation to the rest of the body. At birth, the cord ends at the L3 level. Further postnatal growth results in the cord ultimately ending at L2.

14.038 Which cranial nerve is the lowest numbered cranial nerve arising from the myelencephalon?

A. olfactory nerve - CN I
B. optic nerve - CN II
C. oculomotor nerve - CN III
D. trochlear nerve - CN IV
E. trigeminal nerve - CN V
F. abducens nerve - CN VI
G. facial nerve - CN VII
H. vestibulocochlear nerve - CN VIII
I. glossopharyngeal nerve - CN IX
J. vagus nerve - CN X
K. accessory nerve - CN XI
L. hypoglossal nerve - CN XII

I. is correct.
If you remember 1-1-2-4-4, you will know the pattern of cranial nerves arising from the 5 brain vesicles: telencephalon - I, diencephalon - II, mesencephalon - III, IV, metencephalon - V, VI, VII, VIII, myelencephalon - IX, X, XI, XII.